4/08

D0073011

Natural Treatments for Chronic Fatigue Syndrome

Recent Titles in
Complementary and Alternative Medicine

Herbs and Nutrients for the Mind: A Guide to Natural Brain Enhancers
Chris Demetrois Meletis, N.D. and Jason E. Barker, N.D.

Asperger Syndrome: Natural Steps toward a Better Life
Suzanne C. Lawton, N.D.

Natural Treatments for Chronic Fatigue Syndrome

Daivati Bharadvaj, N.D.

Complementary and Alternative Medicine
Chris D. Meletis, Series Editor

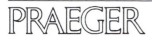

Westport, Connecticut
London

Library of Congress Cataloging-in-Publication Data

Bharadvaj, Daivati.
Natural treatments for chronic fatigue syndrome / Daivati Bharadvaj.
     p. ; cm. – (Complementary and alternative medicine, ISSN 1549–084X)
    Includes bibliographical references and index.
    ISBN 978–0–275–99374–0 (alk. paper)
    1. Chronic fatigue syndrome—Alternative treatment.   I. Title.   II. Series:
Complementary and alternative medicine (Westport, Conn.)
[DNLM: 1. Fatigue Syndrome, Chronic—therapy.   2. Naturopathy. WB 146 B575n
2007]
  RB150.F37B52   2008
  616′.0478–dc22   2007038901

British Library Cataloguing in Publication Data is available.

Library of Congress Catalog Card Number: 2007038901
ISBN: 0–275–99374–4
ISSN: 1549–084X

First published in 2008

Praeger Publishers, 88 Post Road West, Westport, CT 06881
An imprint of Greenwood Publishing Group, Inc.
www.praeger.com

Printed in the United States of America

The paper used in this book complies with the
Permanent Paper Standard issued by the National
Information Standards Organization (Z39.48–1984).

10 9 8 7 6 5 4 3 2 1

To my teachers and mentors,
who have taught me the art of medicine;

and

to my patients,
who teach me everyday how to be a better doctor.

Contents

Series Foreword

More than 1 million people suffer from chronic fatigue syndrome, meeting all the diagnostic criteria. In addition, some 10 million people in the United States suffer some but not all the symptoms, with their lives just as dramatically impacted and compromised. And chronic fatigue is an equal opportunity condition, affecting people of every age, gender, ethnicity, and socioeconomic group. Women face a higher incidence than men, and this condition is more prevalent in people in their 40s and 50s, though it can affect people of all ages, young and old alike.

Dr. Daivati Bharadvaj and the growing number of physicians that embrace health care from a truly integrative approach are pioneering the way for the next quantum leap in significant advances in both academic and clinical medicine. With the support of the National Institutes of Health (NIH) and National Center for Complementary and Alternative Medicine (NCCAM), and funding from both private and public sectors, the appreciation for the integration of health-care education and delivery is becoming greater.

This is a pivotal time for all health-care providers to embrace the concept of "individualized patient oriented wellness." Thanks to the work of Dr. David Eisenberg and similar researchers, we now know that Americans are allocating billions of discretionary dollars to seek out what used to be termed as "alternative medicine" approaches. Yet what was once considered fully "alternative" is becoming integrated, as evidence grows, into the mainstream.

This book on Chronic Fatigue Syndrome is an important contribution that provides a platform for health-care provider and patient alike to proceed with a heightened level of awareness and insight. It offers a head start in establishing a working foundation to meet the unique needs of patients as they participate in the lifelong health-care journey, which should be, with the advent of an integrated approach, more accurately termed "wellness care." We must applaud

Dr. Bharadvaj, and all healthcare providers willing to delve into the medical research on the quest to provide hope and inspiration for those challenged with health conditions that are all too often either ignored or lack adequate traditional treatment options.

Chris D. Meletis, N.D.
Series Editor, Complementary and Alternative Medicine

Acknowledgments

I wish to thank my family and friends and colleagues for all of their blessings; they make me joyous and inspired to do great things every day. Special appreciation to my parents, Devi and Satish, and my brother, Akar, who are always by my side and who have given me a solid foundation of support and unconditional love; to Kevin for reminding me to be young at heart; to my friends who keep me going no matter what hardship comes; to Dr. Chris Meletis for planting the seed in my head and offering mentorship throughout the writing process; to Tami Dunstan who inspired me to study this condition in the first place; to Taunya Jernigan for her amazing illustrations, and for her ability to be objective and keep things light; to Rick Severson and the library staff at the National College of Naturopathic Medicine for all of their help in acquiring journal articles; to my fellow practitioners at Jade River Healing Arts Center for their encouragement and belly laughs; and of course to all the researchers, physicians, scientists all around the world for their hard work and exploration into the basis of natural medicines. They provide the fresh scientific understanding and pioneering perspective that keep the field of natural medicine progressing and evolving.

Introduction

Tami seems happier than I have ever seen her. She stands confidently in the sunshine, her long white gown ruffling in the breeze. It is not just the fact that she is a bride on her wedding day that makes her beautiful. She actually has radiance about her, in her face, in her step, and especially in her laughter. And it is very inspiring to see her in this way.

A few years ago, Tami first came to see me for her long-term debilitating fatigue. It seemed to start 13 years prior, just after a bout with a serious flu with characteristics of infectious mononucleosis. Even at that time, no one had tested her for antibodies against viruses and other pathogens or evaluated her for complex symptoms. Tami's energy was always very low. She needed excessive amounts of sleep and still never really felt refreshed during the day. Not only did she "hit a wall" with her exercise, but she also experienced excessive muscle pain and inflexibility. This made it difficult for her to hold her career as a personal fitness trainer. She also had a history of allergies and skin sensitivity as a child, and endometriosis and recurrent infections as an adult.

She was told by every other health care professional that "it's all in your head" and that there was nothing really wrong with her, therefore there was nothing that could be done. After doing a diagnostic workup for chronic fatigue syndrome (CFS), we found elevated levels of EBV and HHV viral antibody titers in her blood, abnormally high levels of lymphocytes, and imbalanced hormones such as estrogen, DHEA, and cortisol. We ruled out other medical conditions that appear to cause symptoms of weakness and chronic fatigue, and finally agreed that she met the criteria for CFS with viral origin, immune dysfunction, and neuroendocrine imbalance. She, like many others, seemed relieved to have her health concerns validated and given a real definition. Now she had somewhere to go.

Within a few months of starting regular IV nutrient therapy, antiviral and immune-modulating herbal medicines, and hormone-balancing nutritional supplements, Tami starting noticing significant improvement in her energy levels and outlook on life. She started to "feel normal again." After about 1 year of regular therapy and compliance with a healthy diet with nutritional and herbal supplements she claimed that this was "the best [she] felt in 15 years!"

We could easily attribute her success story to the natural medicines she was using. But really, Tami found her own cure. Given the nourishment, rest, and support for recovery, her body's own natural healing processes jumpstarted. Her energy returned slowly but steadily, and she could soon resume doing all of the activities she once really enjoyed. She was able to thrive in her practice as a fitness trainer, regain her own physical fitness, and start school to become certified in the field of real estate. She stopped losing hair, gained some musculature, and started looking more vibrant. Even her sassy attitude started to return, and pretty soon her personality was itself contagious! It was as if she found her inner spirit all over again.

Tami's story, and the stories of others who have sought my help for similar health concerns, continues to inspire me to research, study, and learn more about this enigmatic condition called CFS. There is an abundance of new material in the medical literature discussing clinical data and scientific evidence, as well as a variety of intriguing theories to explain how these different concepts come together. And while the current medical pharmaceutical model of treatment lacks real solutions for people suffering from this condition, there are plenty of natural medicines that can and do offer safe and effective treatment options.

This book is based on scientific evidence, medical research, and the thousands of years of clinical wisdom passed down from natural medicine traditions from around the world. CFS can be a complicated condition in that this illness affects every level of functioning in the body, across multiple organ systems. Because of this, it is vital to approach the understanding and treatment of this condition from many angles, including mind, body, spirit, and lifestyle influences. We need to address CFS from a comprehensive holistic perspective for the therapy to be successful, and for each individual inflicted with this condition to find his/her own personal healing journey through the process. It is my goal to share all of the information I have gleaned with those who might really benefit from it. In this way, I hope that others who suffer from CFS can use the medical understanding, physician support, and their own inner healing ability to overcome their illness.

PART I

What Is Chronic Fatigue Syndrome?

CHAPTER 1

Concepts, Controversies, and Conventional Medicine

HISTORY

Few conditions have received as much controversial attention as chronic fatigue syndrome (CFS). Debates commenced from the very beginning. In the early stages of its "discovery," the medical community had trouble combining this complex of seemingly unrelated symptoms, and the question of whether CFS was truly its own "organic" disease evoked confusion. That being the case, CFS was lumped into categories such as neurasthenia,[1] myalgic encephalomyelitis, and even psychiatric disorders.[2] When CFS finally established its own identity, there was much disagreement about defining something so indeterminate, while some refuted its very existence.[3] Fortunately, CFS did attract attention from many researchers and clinicians, who began to figure out what caused this complex disorder, how to diagnose it, how to distinguish it from other disorders, and of course, how to treat a person affected by it.

In 1994, a fundamental definition for CFS had emerged.[4] And in 2003, this case definition was revised to exclude psychiatric illness.[5] CFS was presented as a condition of long-lasting fatigue with no relief, accompanied by other mental, emotional, and physical symptoms of no other origin. Creating a definition provided a solid starting point from which to go forward. The first step was to recognize that the problem with a basic definition is, in itself, "basic." Some questions that remained unanswered were: How many people continue to be affected? What diagnostic tests can we rely on? How do we know if therapy is truly effective? How will the very definition of CFS evolve in light of new research?

Around this time, despite our definitions, the Centers for Disease Control (CDC) had concluded that "no pathognomonic tests have been validated in scientific studies"[6] to diagnose CFS. This meant that we did not have a surefire way to figure out if someone truly had CFS or if that individual "just feels tired." It also presented a challenge for health care providers to differentiate CFS from somatoform diseases, mental disorders with physical symptoms lacking an organic cause.

In light of many recent clinical treatments and outcome studies, the CDC has also implied that "no definitive treatments exist" and most people with CFS will "remain functionally impaired for years."[6] And yet, there is so much to be optimistic about. Contrary to earlier thought, CFS sufferers may now seek support from natural therapeutics with documented treatment outcomes and continued clinical research trials. Scientific evidence reveals specific disease patterns, trends, risk factors, diagnostic parameters, and other measurements to evaluate people with possible chronic fatigue. The emergence of evidence-based medical literature and human clinical trials gives credit to the variety of different natural treatments for CFS honored in "alternative" healing medical traditions from around the world.

So where do we go from here? On the one hand, while given all the controversy over definitions, risk factors, diagnostic criteria, and effective therapies for CFS, it is little wonder that so much attention has been given to this health topic. On the other hand, with all the media and public intrigue, we still need continued research and discussion to better understand this disorder. We can only improve our comprehension, our acceptance of the intricacies of this condition, based on our next steps.

SYMPTOMS AND COMPLEXITIES OF OVERLAP WITH OTHER CONDITIONS

Recently, in 2003, CFS experts reached consensus for a more accurate definition of this condition. The proposed newer definition, which completely excluded psychiatric disorders, both confirmed and supported the original 1994 definition characterized by severe fatigue. Unfortunately for linear thinkers, a definition based on symptoms (subjective information which patients report) instead of lab results or physical signs (objective information which most clinicians and scientists adore) presents an unclear description which in turn creates more confusion. Nevertheless, to be diagnosed with CFS, a person would need to suffer from fatigue lasting more than 6 months, which cannot be relieved with rest. This fatigue must dramatically reduce the person's ability to handle previous work and personal activities. Additionally, CFS manifests physically by causing concentration difficulties, sore throats and tender lymph nodes, muscle pain, headaches, and sleep disorders. People with these problems need not have other medical conditions to explain them, nor should they have psychiatric disorders, substance abuse, eating disorders, or severe obesity.

Symptoms of this condition can be grouped according to major and minor criteria for diagnosing CFS, according to the Centers for Disease Control and Prevention (CDC),[7] summarized in Table 1.1. Major criteria simply require that an individual suffers from new onset of fatigue causing 50 percent reduction

Table 1.1. CDC & P Diagnostic Criteria for Chronic Fatigue Syndrome

Major Criteria
- New onset of fatigue causing 50% reduction in activity for at least 6 months
- Exclusion of other illnesses that can cause fatigue

Minor Criteria

Presence of eight of the eleven symptoms listed below, or six of the eleven symptoms and two of the three signs

Symptoms
1. Mild fever
2. Recurrent sore throat
3. Painful lymph nodes
4. Muscle weakness
5. Muscle pain
6. Prolonged fatigue after exercise
7. Recurrent headache
8. Migratory joint pain
9. Neurologic or psychologic complaints
   - Sensitivity to bright light
   - Forgetfulness
   - Confusion
   - Inability to concentrate
   - Excessive irritability
   - Depression
10. Sleep disturbance (hypersomnia or insomnia)
11. Sudden onset of symptom complex

Signs
1. Low-grade fever
2. Nonexudative pharyngitis
3. Palpable or tender lymph nodes

in activity for at least 6 months, and that no other illness that causes fatigue explains the nature of this individual's fatigue. Minor criteria include a wider range of symptoms and clinical signs. The presence of either eight of the eleven symptoms listed, or six of the eleven symptoms plus two of the three signs, is diagnostic for CFS:

Symptoms:
1. mild fever
2. recurrent sore throat
3. painful lymph nodes
4. muscle weakness
5. muscle pain
6. prolonged fatigue after exercise
7. recurrent headache

8. migratory joint pain
9. neurological or psychological complains such as sensitivity to bright light, forgetfulness, confusion, inability to concentrate, excessive irritability, and depression
10. sleep disturbance (hypersomnia or insomnia)
11. sudden onset of symptom complex.

Signs:
1. low-grade fever
2. nonexudative pharyngitis
3. palpable or tender lymph nodes.

Table 1.2 reveals the frequency of other symptoms found in this condition. Apparently, CFS is not just about chronic fatigue. In fact, some of these other mental, emotional, or physical complaints may be just as prominent as fatigue. In addition to the already-mentioned symptoms, patients may also report concomitant issues such as gastrointestinal disturbances, dizziness, nausea, change of appetite, and night sweats.[8] Naming chronic fatigue a "syndrome" allows these complexities and nuances to be fully embraced.

The very nature of fatigue itself may be quite different in CFS. People with CFS have acute onset, or sudden, fatigue, whereas people without CFS endure a gradual progression of fatigue with some amelioration from rest and the wonderful ability to recover.

Many people seem to have concomitant, or simultaneous, psychiatric disorders with CFS. This may be due to overlapping definitions for both illnesses.[3] Of course a person with CFS might also suffer from depressive episodes or other psychological symptoms as a normal reaction to the physical illness. The one major distinction between depression and CFS, however, is that CFS patients generally do not respond to antidepressant medications.[9] Interestingly, certain psychological and behavioral therapies (such as cognitive behavior therapy) can be effective in people with CFS whether or not they also suffer from psychiatric disorders. Thus, perhaps some CFS patients may suffer from mental-emotional disorders which are clearly distinct from psychiatric disorders all together. Table 1.3 describes the conditions that would exclude the diagnosis of CFS despite overlap in symptomatology.

PREVALENCE

While fatigue remains the single most common symptom driving people to seek medical care, only a small percentage of those fatigued individuals actually have CFS. According to one review in the United States, "24% of the general adult population has experienced fatigue lasting 2 weeks or longer, with 59% to 64% of these people reporting no medical cause."[10] Up to one-quarter of primary care clinic patients reported having had prolonged fatigue lasting around 1 month.[11] But to be defined as chronic fatigue, this symptom needs to last beyond 6 months.[12]

Table 1.2. Frequency of Symptoms in CFS

Symptom/sign	Frequency (%)
Fatigue	100
Low-grade fever	60–95
Muscle pain	20–95
Sleep disorder	15–90
Impaired mental function	50–85
Depression	70–85
Headache	35–85
Allergies	55–80
Sore throat	50–75
Anxiety	50–70
Muscle weakness	40–70
Postexercise fatigue	50–60
Premenstrual syndrome (women)	50–60
Stiffness	50–60
Visual blurring	50–60
Nausea	50–60
Dizziness	30–50
Joint pain	40–50
Dry eyes and mouth	30–40
Diarrhea	30–40
Cough	30–40
Decreased appetite	30–40
Night sweats	30–40
Painful lymph nodes	30–40

1. Clinically evaluated, unexplained, persistent, or relapsing fatigue for at least 6 months that:
   - Is of new or definite onset
   - Is not the result of ongoing exertion
   - Is not substantially alleviated by rest
   - Results in substantial reduction in previous levels of occupational, educational, social, or personal activities
2. Four or more of the following concurrent symptoms on a persistent or recurrent basis during 6 or more consecutive months of illness, none of which may predate the fatigue.
   - Self-reported impairment in short-term memory or concentration that is severe enough to cause substantial reduction in previous levels of occupational, educational, social, or personal activities
   - Sore throat
   - Tender cervical or axillary lymph nodes
   - Muscle pain
   - Multijoint pain without joint swelling or redness
   - Headaches of a new type, pattern, or severity
   - Unrefreshing sleep
   - Postexertional malaise lasting more than 24 hours

Both 1 and 2 are required conditions for a diagnosis of CFS

Table 1.3. Conditions that Exclude the Diagnosis of CFS

- Any active medical condition that may explain the presence of chronic fatigue (e.g., untreated hypothyroidism, sleep apnea, narcolepsy, adverse effects of medications, HIV disease)
- Any previously diagnosed medical condition without resolution documented beyond reasonable clinical doubt, and **for which** continued activity may explain the chronic fatiguing illness, (e.g., previously **treated** malignancies and unresolved cases of hepatitis B or hepatitis C virus infection)
- Any past or current diagnosis of major depression with melancholic or psychotic features, bipolar affective disorder, schizophrenia of any subtype, delusional disorders of any subtype, dementias of any type, anorexia nervosa, or bulimia
- Alcohol or other substance abuse within 2 years before the onset of the chronic fatigue and any time afterward
- Severe obesity as defined by a body mass index (BMI) ≥ 45:

$$BMI = \frac{\text{weight in kg}}{(\text{height in m})^2}$$

- Any unexplained physical examination finding or laboratory or imaging test abnormality that strongly suggests the presence of an exclusionary condition

A main distinguishing point is that people with CFS suffer from more severe psychological distress and, therefore, tend to consult their providers more frequently.[13] Also, they are twice as likely to suffer from depression and more than twice as likely to be unemployed. People with CFS tend to have other related symptoms such as sleep disorders, pain, concentration difficulties, and sore throats. So while most of the population is affected by fatigue at some point, those with CFS suffer quite a bit more.

Earlier studies by the CDC estimated a minimum of 4.6 to 11.3 per 100,000 people were affected with CFS in 1993.[14] Surveys distributed in four major U.S. cities from 1989 to 1993 found lower prevalence rates but gathered that most people with CFS were white women with the average age of 30.[15] Almost all had completed high school and more than 1/3 graduated from college. The mean household income for these people was $40,000. It was starting to look like CFS primarily affected young white working women. The authors concluded that "education and income levels might have influenced usage of the health-care system, and the populations of these four surveillance sites might not be representative of the U.S. population." To follow up, they concentrated on just one surveillance site, Wichita, Kansas, and found prevalence rates to be much higher (235 out of 100,000 or 2.35%) and concluded that CFS was a "major public health problem."[16]

For a while, because of the higher prevalence among young educated urbanites, CFS was nicknamed the "yuppie flu." But the chronically fatigued young white working class myth was soon busted in 1998 when a San Fransisco study found elevated CFS rates among African Americans as well as Native Americans.[17] The rates were lower in Asian minority groups. Prevalence rates were 0.2 percent of the general population for CFS-like illness. Again, more women were affected than men, the average income was below $40,000, and people in clerical occupations were more likely to be affected. Studying a more diverse population (such as that of San Francisco) allows researchers to glean a more complete background about people from different socioeconomic levels and minority groups. In this case, results show that CFS is not selective for class or race or even gender; it affects people of various backgrounds.

Interesting epidemiological findings started emerging. In the Pacific Northwest, not only did people with CFS have poorer functional status and higher rates of psychological distress, but they more commonly had enlarged or swollen cervical (neck) or axillary (underarm) lymph nodes.[18] This study supported a prevalence rate of up to 267/100,000 people affected with CFS. In Iceland, up to 1.4 percent of the population was classified with CFS.[19] The average age of 44 was higher than that in the United States, and the authors found some correlations between CFS and phobias or panic disorders. In 2004, an adolescent-based study determined lower CFS rates in teens than that in adults.[20] Not surprisingly, "significant differences existed between parental and adolescents' descriptions of illness," suggesting the importance of interviewing the person affected, and possible lack of communication between the teens and their parents about personal health issues.

According to a *Lancet* review in 2006, prevalence rates in the United States were 0.23 and 0.42 percent per two different studies.[21] These studies also found that CFS seemed to affect women more than men, although perhaps women were simply being diagnosed more often due to the higher likelihood of seeking medical care for their fatigue. Regardless, CFS also seemed to affect people with "lower educational attainment and occupational status." The rates were also higher among minority groups, especially minority women, in the United States. The prevalence seemed a bit higher in the United Kingdom, and other nations, where the rates were found to be in the range of 2 to 3 percent of the population. The differences in rates may be attributable to differences in study methods or definition used.

While it is likely that at least two million U.S. adults suffer from CFS,[22] discrepancies in the designs of these studies reflect some of the inconsistent findings. The use of different case definitions leads to a wide range of prevalence rates. Including a diversity of regions and population subtypes in these studies provides more information about how CFS may be affecting people living in rural areas or people in different minority groups or those from differing levels of socioeconomic status. In addition, although many studies have found higher rates in women, this may be partially attributed to the lower rates of men seeking medical care in general. We can move past the idea of CFS affecting only urban white women and "yuppies." Also, we can propose that some who were unavailable to be evaluated for CFS after turning in surveys might have indeed met the criteria for this condition. The authors of the 2006 Lancet review suggest that since "very little reliable" or "valid" data exist, future studies need to address prevalence in the general public rather than in specialty centers. Probably, even the higher estimates of 522 women and 291 men per 100,000 may still be conservative,[23] and future research may find that more than 2.2 million Americans are affected with CFS.

FACTORS THAT CONTRIBUTE TO DEVELOPMENT OF CFS

For a long time, the majority of studies focused on physical causes of CFS. More recent studies have started addressing mental-emotional factors as well. While many ideas are proposed (viral infections, neurological dysfunction, psychological factors, hormonal imbalances, and even personality traits), only a few of these explanations are confirmed in multiple studies.[21] In general, CFS is said to be a multifactorial disease, one in which many factors integrate together to create the symptoms.

A person's vulnerability to CFS may be related to her personality. Apparently, having "introverted" or "neurotic" tendencies increases the likelihood of developing this condition.[24] Both introversion and neuroses are characterized by avoidant behavior and anxiety. In addition, CFS tends to run among families, with a possible genetic predisposition.[25] Being female also presents a higher risk. So does being inactive as a child, or being lethargic after being sick from infectious mononucleosis.[26] It is a wonder that more people do not develop CFS for these reasons.

Several outside factors can trigger the onset of CFS. Many people report never feeling well since an infection such as a flu or infectious mono. Others begin descending into chronic fatigue after infections with Lyme disease or Epstein-Barr virus.[27] Life-altering events—serious injury, stress, trauma, surgery, grief, loss and bereavement, and even pregnancy and labor[28]—may precipitate this disorder. In this way, CFS mimics posttraumatic stress disorder or PTSD.

Studies are finding that some perpetuating factors reduce chance of recovery for people who already have CFS.[29] Family members and friends and even health-care providers can enable a person's negative outlook by dwelling on illness instead of on possible recovery. Some people suffering from CFS find it difficult to imagine full recovery. Perhaps they have suffered too long and have lost hope. Perhaps they are not familiar with a more functional life after suffering. And recovery might mean renouncing the special attention and care they received with the hated label of illness, which they have become dependent on. In one study, this "solicitous behavior" even afforded financial benefits to some who were deeply affected with CFS.[29] There may be hidden blessings that come with being ill at the cost of optimal wellness.

Surprisingly, functional impairment may not have much to do with actual physical fatigue. The former seems more related to the perception of ability to function. In fact, negative perception may be the true cause of inactivity and avoidant behavior, according to one study.[30] Loss of hope and obsession over physical body sensations can further impair functioning. The feelings of disempowerment which come with negative perception are not necessarily unfounded however. Many people dealing with CFS experience lack of support from loved ones and also from health-care providers who fail to acknowledge the diagnosis and severity of this condition. It is important to avoid "blaming the victim" by acknowledging the situation for what it is while working with the individual to understand and support his needs.

MECHANISMS AND DIAGNOSIS

Possible mechanisms for developing CFS are just as varied and unclear as any other aspect of this condition. Overall, there are three main conventional understandings of the pathophysiology—neuroendocrine, immunological dysfunction, and central nervous system disorder. Research has shown evidence of a neuroendocrine pathway explaining the connection between stress hormones and CFS symptoms.[31] Despite being challenged with hormones to stimulate the stress response, many people with CFS have a lower than normal cortisol reaction. Cortisol is a hormone produced in the adrenal glands above the kidneys to mount a survival reaction to physical, mental, or emotional stressors. Without sufficient cortisol, the body shuts down in the presence of external stressful events. Perhaps this burning out is what feels like unrecoverable fatigue to CFS sufferers.

Another biological mechanism for CFS is based on immune system dysfunction. Many studies show that people with CFS have higher than average levels of immune cells and components including interleukins and cytokines, chemicals involved in inflammation and immune reactions during illness or injury. In fact, high levels of one of the interleukins, IL-6, may be responsible for "sickness behavior" symptoms such as apathy, sleepiness, loss of appetite, inability to maintain focus or concentration, and heightened pain sensitivity.[32] Interestingly, many of these same symptoms are found in people suffering from depression, making this a potential link between the physical and mental aspects of CFS.

Finally, there may be a clear disturbance on the level of the central nervous system or the brain. In MRI (magnetic resonance imaging) studies, certain areas of the brain were activated during "erroneous performance" of motor imagery tasks, indicating what the authors described as "motivational disturbance."[33] In other words, specific regions of the brain might not be functioning optimally. The same scientists also found that people with CFS had reduced volumes of grey matter in the brain. This likely does not affect mental capacity but only influences functioning and perception in the brain.

When it comes to a common protocol for diagnosing CFS, not surprisingly, the scientific medical community lacks one. Again, there are many difficulties in making an accurate diagnosis. Some patients may present to their physicians having already given themselves the CFS label based on their own knowledge or understanding. Others may not be able to comprehend why they are experiencing these symptoms at all. Some may misuse their fatigue symptoms to claim insurance or disability benefits, or just attention from medical professionals. Others may correlate their CFS symptoms entirely to a preexisting condition, never bothering to question or evaluate their fatigue. Providers are challenged with finding ways to support people in any of these scenarios, juggling a delicate balance between dismissing the fatigue altogether and overplaying a symptom that may or may not be a real issue. Some practitioners disqualify health problems if diagnostic tests cannot confirm abnormal findings, not realizing that CFS is mostly a subjective illness, one that cannot be tested out.

All in all, it becomes difficult to accurately diagnose a condition based on vague subjective parameters. Most of the diagnostic criteria for CFS can be assessed just from a comprehensive patient history. The use of a questionnaire to ascertain fatigue severity may be a reliable and necessary tool. Following a thorough history-taking, physical examination and basic laboratory testing are required to rule out underlying conditions. Since research has not pointed to a specific diagnostic test for CFS, these lab tests would only serve to detect other conditions causing fatigue.[34] Of course, it is entirely possible for an individual to suffer from CFS as well as other conditions simultaneously. A person being treated for these other conditions who experienced persistent fatigue might need to be evaluated for CFS as well.

The most important aspect about diagnosis, aside from accuracy, is giving a person the chance to talk about her health concerns and acknowledge her suffering as true and valid to her. In a way, a proper diagnosis can only be made based on understanding the individual, not merely the labeling the condition he presents with. The art of listening without passing judgment can in itself provide clues to successful treatment by establishing the trust and communication so vital to good treatment outcomes. Rapport between doctor and patient not only prevents mishaps and setbacks but it may be at the very core of true healing.

CONVENTIONAL TREATMENTS AND FUTURE EXPLORATION

So far, conventional treatments for CFS primarily revolve around psychological and physical medicine. A 2006 Lancet journal review article showcased Cognitive Behavior Therapy (CBT) and Graded Exercise Therapy (GET) as the most effective treatment options for people with CFS.[21] Several researchers on CBT propose that this treatment can help guide people to "acquire control" over their symptoms. As perception of disempowerment is one of the perpetuating factors of CFS, it makes sense that a psychological approach toward empowerment would be effective. In CBT, people are challenged to form new cognitive patterns while letting go of former ways of thinking. Reconditioning the mind's habit response enables a person to stop reacting in the same ways while opening up to alternative, more effective responses.

GET offers physical rehabilitation by using a graded physical activity program. This allows people with CFS to achieve a reasonable goal, maintain that level of activity, and then increase to the next goal in increments. With each achievement a person gains a sense of empowerment and hope to strive for continued physical aptitude. Even though GET does not aim to address the mental-emotional aspects of CFS, it still shows a 55 percent rate of improvement. CBT boasts a near 70 percent improvement rate by successfully addressing the cognitive aspects.

According to this same article, studies evaluating the use of corticosteroid-based pharmaceutical medications for CFS were deemed "inconclusive," or failing to provide sufficient evidence of efficacy.[21] Another study found that the use of antihistamines and medications to slow down the immune system response to allergies and CFS-related immune dysfunction was also ineffective.[35] Using immunologic medicines combined with psychologic approaches also failed to demonstrate clinical benefit.[36] Despite the immune dysfunction characteristic of CFS, treatment using intravenous immunoglobulin therapy has not been recommended.[37] Even the antibiotic approach to destroying certain microorganisms considered responsible for triggering CFS seems unuseful.[38] While conventional medicine continues to search for medicines and other answers to treat those suffering from CFS, there are a variety of positive treatment outcomes with using nutrients and herbal medicines instead. Using the framework of many alternative medicine models provides a way to view the "whole picture," including all of the complexities of this condition as well as the uniqueness of each individual suffering from this condition.

Newer medical research models are expanding ways of studying and evaluating treatments regarding CFS. Using a biopsychosocial model for studying CFS resolves the old conflict between psychology and physiology. This model integrates the biological, psychological, and social factors present in this illness. So the debate over CFS being either psychogenic (mental) or somatic (physical) in nature can finally lay to rest. Scientists have already started to look at how neurobiology correlates with psychology. This allows health-care providers to explain to their patients why the condition is "not all in your head." Now health care workers and patients alike can observe the totality of the different features of this illness enabling us to use a more holistic perspective.

Although some suggest that there is "insufficient evidence" to support the effectiveness of complementary interventions,[21] there is in fact a rising body of evidence showing the efficacy of various natural medicine modalities. Clinical research is supporting the use of nutrition, diet therapy, botanical medicines, homeopathy, and other interventions in the treatment of people with CFS. To modern science and medical practice this condition may seem relatively new. Yet we can trace back to traditional medicines around the globe to search for answers on what worked then, and what might work now. For example, long before CFS was even considered a real condition, people were successfully treating similar conditions of severe fatigue with the ancient wisdom of Ayurvedic and Chinese medicines. Today we can explore those protocols, continue the clinical research, and enhance what knowledge we already have about natural treatments for CFS.

CHAPTER 2

Etiologies

OVERVIEW

Where does CFS come from? Like many diseases, chronic fatigue syndrome (CFS) has multiple causes and a checkered history. In the mid-1700s, CFS was called the "little fever" to describe the symptoms of weariness, forgetfulness, pain, and low-grade fever.[1] A century later, it was termed neurasthenia due to the profound fatigue which was thought to be from "lack of nerve strength."[2] Around the same time, a physician-researcher observed Civil War soldiers suffering from fatigue, chest pain, dizziness, sleep difficulties, and heart palpitations which he linked to "irritable heart."[3] This condition later became appropriately known as the "effort syndrome."[4] Although the popularity of this label wore off after a few decades, other similar conditions kept arising in reports for a long time. While the name and theorized causative factors of CFS have evolved, there may still be some relevance and significance to the previous ideas about this condition.

For as many titles that it has had, CFS has had at least as many purported causes. No one single cause has been completely accepted in medical practice and scientific understanding yet today. Many long-running theories have been refuted in scientific review articles. Microorganisms like Brucella, Candida (yeast), Borrelia (the Lyme disease-causing spirochete), herpes viruses,[5] and human retroviruses have all remained unproven in the medical literature as possible pathogenic causes of CFS.[6] This means that no one has definitively stated how much (if at all) these microorganisms play a role in the establishment or development of CFS. The chronic Epstein-Barr virus infection (EBV) has been thought to be the main culprit for a long time[7] but even it is being refuted by some studies.[8] Other potential causes have not yet been fully substantiated, nor ruled out. Current research reveals connections to allergies and atopic conditions,[9] immune

Table 2.1. Pathogenesis of CFS

Predisposing factors that increase likelihood of acquiring CFS	Precipitating factors that trigger the onset of CFS	Perpetuating factors that worsen symptoms and course of illness
Psychiatric illness	Infection	Reduced physical fitness
Genetic	Stress and negative life events	Concurrent psychiatric illness
Environment (e.g., allergy, chemicals, toxins)	Immune system dysfunction	Misattribution of physical symptoms
	Oxidative stress and mitochondrial damage	Raised immunomodulating chemicals such as cytokines

abnormalities, nutritional deficiencies, abnormal endocrine or hormonal responses to stress, mitochondrial oxidative stress, and many others causes for CFS. It is likely that many of these issues exacerbate one another, leading to the condition as a whole. Table 2.1 reviews the predisposing factors that increase likelihood of developing CFS, precipitating factors that trigger the onset, and perpetuating factors that worsen the course of illness.

IMMUNE SYSTEM DYSFUNCTIONS

The immune system provides the body the ability to recognize and fight off foreign substances, which might otherwise cause harm. Upon injury, an array of immune cells and chemicals set out to destroy and dispose of any foreign materials (also called antigens). Immune cells called T lymphocytes are responsible for long-term recognition and destruction of antigens, using chemicals to decompose anything which does not belong in the human body. T lymphocytes are composed of helper cells (CD4) to recruit other immune factors, and cytotoxic cells (CD8) to destroy pathogens such as bacteria and viruses. Another type of immune cell, the B lymphocyte, is designed to build specific antibodies to react to those unique antigens. Antibodies are examples of immunoglobulins, immune cell proteins that can specifically recognize antigens and start the immune reaction. There are many other immunological factors including natural killer cells (NK cells) to release chemicals that destroy foreign substances, cytokines to enhance inflammation, and a myriad of proteins to optimize removal of wastes. The immune system creates very complex and intricate ways for the body to protect itself from harm.

The last two decades of research show various unique immune abnormalities associated with CFS. Starting in the late 1980s, studies have been pointing to substantial differences in both populations of specific immune cells as well as immune functioning between people with CFS and healthy control groups. In one study, not only did people with CFS have significantly lower numbers of T lymphocytes (including both helper and cytotoxic cells), but they also had reduced T cell function as evidenced by delayed hypersensitivity skin testing.

In addition, more than half of the CFS group had lower total immunoglobulin levels compared to the healthy group.[10] To reflect the immunological aspect of this condition, CFS has more recently taken on yet another name: CFIDS (chronic fatigue immune dysfunction syndrome). However, since these earlier studies, research has provided other intriguing points to ponder as well.

Several more recent studies have found abnormal changes in NK cells responsible for destroying pathogens. Comprehensive immunological analysis showed in several studies that people with CFS had lower numbers of NK cells as well as markedly reduced NK cell activity.[11,12,13] Using flow cytometry as a way to study these factors found abnormal changes in NK cells with increased activation markers but lower activity.[14] In another study, people with CFS produced higher numbers of NK cells but their cells were unable to destroy tumor cells, rendering them less active.[15] Poorly functioning NK cells may explain the immune system disturbance aspects of CFS symptoms.

There are a few explanations for this issue. Ordinarily, NK cell activity is stimulated by an amino acid called L-arginine. In CFS, L-arginine does not enhance NK cell activity as it does in the healthy population. Researchers suggest that there may be a dysfunction in the way that this amino acid is controlled or affected by a substance called nitric oxide produced by the inner lining of blood vessels. It could be that impairment of nitric oxide-mediated L-arginine leads to reduced function of NK cells.[16] Another explanation is that toxic overload to the system can deplete NK cells, reducing their ability to function. In a study which examined the effects of exposure to toxic chemicals (such as organochlorine pesticides), people exposed to those toxins had very similar presentations to those with CFS who were not exposed. Both groups showed lymphocytic abnormalities in addition to reduction in NK cells. This provokes the question whether toxins may be a causative factor in CFS.[17] Interestingly, these patterns of poorly functioning NK cells and changes in lymphocytes are comparable to those seen in people with "chronic viral reactivation."[15] CFS and viral reactivation syndrome can both cause symptoms that feel like a person has never recovered from the cold. Finally, NK cells of healthy people release protein substances called perforins. These perforins enable lysis or breakdown of the cell membranes of pathogens for effective destruction. In one study, the NK cells of people with CFS had reduced amounts of perforins. Since perforins also serve in immune surveillance, they may be an important marker for testing for CFS.[18] Regardless of mechanism, reduced NK cell activity is tightly linked to symptoms of CFS.

A few studies support an alternative hypothesis. In comparing Gulf War veterans with severe fatigue to civilians with CFS, immune parameters were different. Only severely fatigued veterans showed decreases in NK cells along with increases in T lymphocytes, interferons, and other chemical markers. No such significant immune changes were found in the CFS group. As this seems contrary to the immune dysfunction hypothesis, the authors of this study suggest that immune deficiency may not be a causative factor in CFS.[11] In another study, people with CFS did indeed have abnormal immune cell values but these did not change with treatment. Despite improvements in depression with nonpharmacological therapies, the NK cells and lymphocytes remained about the same as before. In this case, clinical outcomes from treatment of this mental aspect of CFS may not be linked to immune dysfunction.[19] In both these studies, small subsets of the population were tested, and it is clear that we need larger long-term studies to fully establish the importance of NK cell activity in CFS.

T cells, B cells, and other immune factors are also affected in people with CFS. Research is finding higher populations of both CD8 and CD4 T lymphocytes, often with changes in the proportions to one another.[12,13,19] Cytotoxic T cells (CD8) of people with CFS also showed decreased perforin synthesis, just like in NK cells.[18] In addition, there are increased intracellular adhesion molecules on monocytes and increased circulating B cells linked to CFS.[12,14] Research still needs to point out the significance of these factors in CFS.

Cytokines, chemical factors that regulate the immune response, play a very important role in the CFS immune dysfunction. In one study, people with CFS and people with infectious mononucleosis both had elevated levels of interleukins, a type of immune chemical factor.[20] Some of the flu-like symptoms associated with CFS may be caused by elevated levels of cytokines and alpha interferons.[21] CFS triggered by infection of parvovirus B19 shows similar trends in cytokine abnormalities as idiopathic CFS (CFS with unknown cause). This may represent a good model to study the viral-immune aspects of CFS.[22] Another point of interest is the study of cytokine expression during exacerbations and remissions of a latent viral infection, causing flare-ups of physical symptoms and psychological disturbances.[23] Understanding the pattern of symptoms as they relate to changes in immune factors can help aim therapies toward regulating the immune system to reduce the intensity of the condition.

As research has shown, various immune factors are associated with CFS. Some immune factors are reduced, many are elevated, and others show significant changes in their ability to function. A group of scientists have concluded that "60% of the 70 CFS individuals studied had elevation of at least one immune mediator."[24] The concept of immune "deficiency" leading to CFS is clearly a misnomer. Instead, it seems more appropriate to view it as immune dysfunction. Several CFS experts even propose the idea of immune activation as part of the pathogenesis of this condition.[21,25] Because many types of immune cells are activated during CFS, researchers have termed this the "polycellular activation" model.[24] One group of scientists studying people with CFS have identified over one hundred genes with "striking differences in expression," most of which were involved in the immune system.[26] In fact, the patterns of immune cell activation seen in people with CFS are similar to those seen in the resolution phase of many acute viral infections[27] and viral reactivation syndrome.[15] As our understanding deepens, we may be able to use trends in immune cells activation and dysfunction as diagnostic patterns for CFS.

Several studies are providing new insights into how immune abnormalities are closely related to specific mental and emotional aspects of CFS. For example, a study compared people with conditions related to toxic exposure (such as organochlorine pesticide toxicity, sick building syndrome, and Gulf War syndrome) to people with CFS without toxic exposure. After appropriate clinical examination and neuropsychological, immunologic, and neuroendocrine tests, the authors determined that hypothalamic disturbance and immune dysfunction were similar in both groups.[17] Hypothalamic disturbance could explain some of the psychoneurological symptoms commonly found in CFS. This potential role of environmental toxicity as a contributor to CFS needs to be further evaluated. Another group of researchers propose that one aspect of immune dysfunction has to do with monocytes, and that these monocytes are reacting to endogenous opioids, the naturally formed chemicals in the human body which induce pain relief and mood changes.[28] It will be interesting to observe how future research reveals the connections between moods, pain, and immune cell function in CFS.

Delving further into the mental-emotional aspects of CFS, there is an equally fascinating association between the brain and the immune system. A group of women with CFS related to low NK cell activity were checked for cognitive functioning as well as fatigue. They were found to have less vigor, more cognitive impairment, and more daytime dysfunction than women diagnosed with CFS who did not have low NK cell activity. Not surprisingly, the same women performed lower on objective measures of cognitive functioning as well.[29] The exact role that NK cells play on cognitive functioning is still unknown. However, temporary brain damage from previous viral infection in people with CFS might reveal the link between immune abnormalities and psychological disturbance. A viral infection stimulates microglial cells of the brain to induce symptoms of fever, malaise, and sleepiness. If these cells get damaged during glandular fever, pain pathways may become altered[30] leading to heightened pain sensitivity seen in many individuals with CFS. Typical CFS symptoms of fatigue and impaired cognitive function may in fact be related to the effects of immune system changes during infection with a virus.

Viruses and latent viral infections are intimately tied to immune parameters and symptoms of CFS. People with CFS have similar cytokine activity as those with CFS triggered by infection of parvovirus B19.[22] Many people with CFS concurrently have active infection with HHV6 (human herpes virus), which seems to worsen the neurological symptoms and replicate the immunological findings of chronic fatigue.[31] This type of viral infection might be a trigger or perpetuating factor for CFS. And finally, one study found that 95 percent of CFS individuals had higher antibody titers for EBV and coxsackie virus,[32] supporting the evidence of a viral association leading to immune cell changes, triggering CFS.

Abnormalities in immune patterns in CFS have multiple roots and varied clinical associations. Although many suffer from concurrent impairment of NK cell activity, most people with CFS have enhanced or exaggerated immune system activity in general. Examples of this immune dysfunction include alterations in the number and activity levels of cells such as T and B lymphocytes, monocytes, NK cells, and various chemical factors of the immune system. Because of this trend, CFS is being characterized as a condition with polycellular immune dysfunction, as opposed to one of immune deficiency. And these immune cell dysfunctions are intimately tied to symptoms, pathology, and various aspects of CFS.

Viruses and Other Microorganisms

Over the last two decades, scientists have been pursuing various reasons for the complex changes in immunology of people with CFS. Many of these immune dysfunctions appear very similar to those changes occurring during infections due to viruses. Research groups have been searching for evidence of a viral origin to fit together all the pieces of the puzzle. Logically, if a single virus comes forth, then efforts can be made toward antimicrobial therapy as a "cure" for CFS. Yet, like so many aspects of CFS, the knowledge base so far about viruses associated with CFS is controversial and limited.

In the mid-1980s several reports focused on EBV as a leading cause of CFS. EBV is the virus whose infection leads to infectious mononucleosis, a long-lasting condition characterized by flu-like symptoms, severe fatigue, enlarged lymph nodes, and slow recovery. In fact, some believe that EBV never really leaves the system, and that once infected, the virus becomes latent and present for a long time. If the virus becomes activated again later, it can lead to CFS. Several studies showed evidence to this idea. In one study, people with persistent unexplained illnesses were found to have active infections with EBV.[33] In another study, adults with persistent illness and unexplained fatigue were also found to have concurrent EBV infections.[34] A prospective case series in the early 1990s found that people with CFS had "persistently elevated titers" to early antigen, compared to control groups. An elevated titer indicates that the body is still producing antibodies to fight off infection by EBV long after the active infection had subsided. Also, the authors concluded that about half of the people suffering from CFS had never fully recovered from infectious mononucleosis.[35] The information gleaned from these studies begs two questions, "How is chronic fatigue syndrome related to EBV and infectious mononucleosis?" and also "Can we use antibodies to EBV as a marker to study severity and progression of CFS?"

A study in Japan proposed a connection between CFS and chronic EBV infection. People with CFS had significantly higher antibody titers to early antigen complex for EBV. These antibodies arose from immunoglobulins (immune cells) produced to fight off infection from the EBV antigens. The study also found that the higher the titer levels, the worse the fatigue. This showed direct evidence and positive relationship between the immune system's reaction to EBV and severity of symptoms for CFS.[36] Another study compared a group of thirty-five individuals diagnosed with CFS who also met the criteria for chronic or reactivated EBV infection to a similar group of individuals suffering from fatigue who did not meet criteria for CFS or EBV infection. The group with chronic EBV infection and CFS reported an influenza-like illness at the onset of the fatigue. They also had a moderately higher rate of losing jobs and unemployment due to fatigue and a moderately higher rate of improvement in the fatigue from recreational activity.[35] In other words, people with CFS from a chronic EBV infection suffered from increased severity of fatigue, a flu-like illness at the origin of their chronic fatigue, and the ability for symptomatic improvement with exercise. Other symptoms of CFS (mood disorders, anxiety, and somatization disorders) were equally common in both the CFS group and the control group. So again, this supports the idea of a positive correlation between chronic EBV infection and severity of fatigue in CFS.

While EBV and CFS may be correlated according to clinical symptoms, laboratory results do not necessarily support this viral association.[37] In one study, the frequency of isolating EBV in blood or saliva of people with CFS was similar to that in the control group. Therefore, symptomatic improvement and resolution did not produce significant changes in the antibody titers.[38] Another study found evidence to support the higher antibody levels in people with CFS than in control groups but did not find any changes in the levels associated with improved outcomes during follow-up testing. The authors concluded that antibodies to EBV were not a useful measurement in evaluating the course of CFS.[39] Even though infection with EBV has been found to clinically relate to CFS, antibody titers to EBV may not serve as a useful marker to gauge the progression of CFS. This leaves the opportunity to find another laboratory measurement to use as a diagnostic tool.

Aside from EBV, many other microorganisms have been thought to be involved with CFS. In fact, scientists have been investigating the presence of many other viruses, bacteria, spirochetes, and even fungus. So far, "antibody levels of other agents, including arboviruses, cytomegalovirus, human herpesvirus-6, varicella-zoster virus, respiratory viruses (adenovirus, parainfluenza virus types 1, 2 and 3, respiratory syncytial virus), hepatitis viruses, measles virus, *Rickettsia* spp., *Bartonella* spp., *Borrelia burgdorferi*, *Chlamydia* spp. and *Candida albicans*, were not found more frequently in CFS patients than in matched controls."[40] In fact, one author concluded that "although many different infectious agents have been suspected of having an etiologic role in CFS, none qualifies as the sole cause of the illness."[21] This statement seems to knock out many theories and legends about a pathogenic organism responsible for causing CFS.

However, several studies shed a hopeful light on new leads. Back in 1988, a report from the UK found higher levels of enterovirus in the stools of individuals with postviral fatigue syndrome.[41] Another study confirmed those results by finding the presence of enterovirus RNA in muscle biopsies of 20 percent of individuals with CFS compared to none in the control group.[42] Enterovirus is a category of viruses that inhabit the intestines, causing gastrointestinal disturbance such as diarrhea. Although a third research study disputes this point,[43] further research is needed to establish the importance of the correlation between enteroviral infection and CFS.

Another virus may be implicated: the human T cell leukemia lymphoma virus (HTLV-1 and HTLV-2). In fact, HTLV-1 antibodies were detected in about half of the individuals with CFS compared to none in the control group. Also, HTLV-1 and HTLV-2 genetic sequences were found in most adults and even children with CFS but none in controls.[44] So far, no other studies have confirmed or refuted this finding. Unfortunately, no other studies have been published regarding the continued research of this group of viruses.

A few isolated studies name several other causative organisms. In 1959, a study found that CFS can develop after acute infection of brucellosis (a condition of undulating fever and malaise caused by a bacterium from the Brucella species).[45]

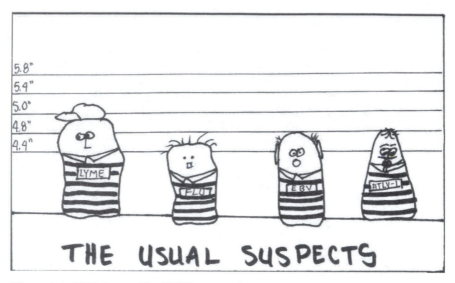

Figure 2.1. EBV, Lyme, Flv, HTLV-1 are "the usual suspects" contributing to CFS development. *Courtesy of Taunya Jernigan.*

Around the same time, another study found that CFS could stem from an acute infection of influenza, or the flu.[46] More recently, one report suggests that CFS may develop after infection of Lyme disease caused by the Borrelia spirochete present in deer ticks, even despite adequate treatment of Lyme disease.[47] Again, these unique studies offer potential for new research to broaden the knowledge base of a pathogenic etiology for CFS.

While no single microorganism can be labeled as the sole cause of CFS, there are a few contenders. Of the few pathogens clearly associated with CFS, only EBV has had several studies to support its positive correlation. Even then, antibody titers to EBV do not seem to be useful markers for diagnosing and evaluating the intensity of the condition. Other pathogens may be similarly related but there is insufficient evidence to make solid conclusions about their involvement in the perpetuation of CFS. As research continues, and the understanding of these pathogens deepens, there may be more information to support a viral (or other microorganism) cause for CFS. For now, all we have are the "usual suspects" that contribute to the development of this disorder (Figure 2.1).

ALLERGIES AND ATOPIC CONDITIONS

Atopy describes the group of conditions, including allergies, asthma, and eczema, which arise from an inappropriate immune response to an otherwise benign substance. A person with atopy will have an inherited hypersensitivity or exaggerated immune response to a substance that would ordinarily evoke no symptoms from a nonatopic individual. Allergies, for example, cause symptoms such as sneezing, itching, redness, discharge, due to the heightened reaction from lymphocytes and IgE immunoglobulins. The idea that CFS may be correlated to allergies and atopy provides more credibility to its immune dysfunction aspect.

Back in 1988, a review article summarizing several areas of research in the field of allergies and CFS proposed that up to 50 percent of individuals with CFS concomitantly had some level of atopy.[48] Since then, another group studied the allergic reactions of individuals tested with metal allergens. Over one hundred individuals (almost half of whom met the criteria for CFS) were patch-tested for eight different metal allergens. Not only did the CFS group show overall increased sensitivity to all the metals, but they also displayed moderately higher levels of nickel allergy than the controls. The nickel allergy seemed to affect women more than men.[49] Perhaps people with CFS are more prone to hypersensitivities, in this case to nickel, due to their predisposing immune dysfunction.

A Barcelona study also demonstrated the prevalence of atopy with CFS. About 30 percent of their CFS individuals studied also had allergic disease. However, the researchers did not find significant symptomatic differences in allergic symptoms from the patients' histories. The inhalant prick tests for allergic reactions to environmental and food allergens also showed no correlation.[50] So even though one-third of the individuals with CFS also had allergies, allergy testing did not seem to provide a way to measure the association between CFS and atopy in this study.

Allergies in people with CFS might be correlated with a type of marker called eosinophilic cationic protein (ECP). In thirty-five individuals with CFS who also suffered from allergies, the levels of ECP were much higher than in healthy individuals who did not have CFS or allergies. Compared to 0 percent of controls, 77 percent of the test group also had a positive RAST test, revealing hypersensitivity to one or more allergens. The RAST test is a common way of evaluating an individual's hypersensitivity to unique allergens. Of the fourteen individuals with CFS who showed higher ECP levels, twelve also showed a positive RAST test. This reveals a correlation between ECP and RAST testing for allergens, as well as the higher prevalence of both in people with CFS. The authors proposed a "common immunologic background" between CFS and atopy.[51] It is yet to be determined exactly what that commonality is, how well it is associated with both conditions, whether one condition predisposes an individual to the other condition, and if there are laboratory markers to test for this association.

Finally, some propose a dysfunction in the relationship between the immunological system and the neuroendocrine system, leading to conditions such as CFS (and even attention deficit hyperactivity disorder ADHD). A dysfunction of the immune system, or hyperactive immune function which triggers allergies, may interface with the neuroendocrine system leading to symptoms of fatigue. Authors of one article explore the idea of food allergies and chronic viral infections as factors that cause both immune and neuroendocrine abnormalities leading to CFS.[52]

Evidence from several scientific studies suggests a relationship between a hyperactive immune response seen in allergic conditions and the prevalence of CFS in individuals with those conditions. It seems uncertain whether immune dysfunction of CFS sets the system up for allergies, or whether an allergic makeup can trigger CFS immune abnormalities. The question that remains is "Exactly how does the presence of allergic immune abnormalities affect the rate of chronic fatigue syndrome?" And if a correlation exists, then further research needs to evaluate possible ways to test for the contribution of atopy to the course of CFS.

Food Intolerances

Allergic reactions to foods and chemicals can cause rashes, itching, hives, sneezing, discharge from the eyes and ears, and other mildly irritating symptoms. In more severe cases, allergies can induce anaphylaxis, a condition where the respiratory passages constrict impairing the individual's ability to breathe. Intolerances, however, are very different. Unlike allergies, they do not evoke the typical pattern of immune system responses to the offensive element. Intolerances to foods and chemicals may take a longer time to set in, causing subtle symptoms at first and more chronic illness later. Typically, most food or chemical intolerances lead to digestive upset, fatigue, subtle mood and behavior fluctuations, joint inflammation and pain, and chronic diseases to name just a few symptoms. It has been suggested that CFS is related to food intolerances.

In one comprehensive medical history questionnaire of 200 individuals with chronic fatigue, many self-reported multiple intolerances to foods.[53] In fact, 13.5 percent of these patients had intolerances to at least three different food groups. Even though physical examination and laboratory testing revealed few abnormalities, those with food intolerances had more functional bodily symptoms. The author of this study attributed this pattern to somatization disorder, a condition where physical symptoms arise from psychogenic illness. However, recent research shows that, more likely, food intolerances are manifestations of the physical dysfunction and symptoms faced by individuals with chronic fatigue.

A review article by Logan and Wong in 2001 cites several studies to support the hypothesis of CFS linked to food intolerances.[54] The authors quote research showing how food intolerances have been related to symptoms such as "headache, myalgia (muscle pain), joint pain, and GI disturbance (digestive upset), symptoms clearly similar to those observed in CFS patients." They also propose the use of an elimination and challenge diet not only as a "gold standard" to diagnose specific troublesome foods per individual person but also as a means toward treatment since this diet has been successful for other illnesses such as "asthma, ulcerative colitis, Crohn's disease, irritable bowel syndrome, and rhinitis."

But what do foods and intolerance to foods have to do with chronic fatigue anyway? It seems that people who eliminate their known food intolerances and then reintroduce those foods evoke an immune reaction. For example, in one study, reducing intake of food intolerances caused a reduction of inflammatory cytokines, chemicals responsible for urging on immune reactions.[55] When provoked with foods containing wheat and dairy, volunteers experienced increased levels of different types of cytokines, along with symptoms characteristic of CFS (fatigue, headaches, muscle and joint pains, and poor digestion). Immune parameters with high cytokine levels have been observed in individuals with CFS.[20,21,25] Both the immune reactions as well as the symptomatic changes from this elimination–provocation diet show similarities to CFS.

Several other studies support this idea. Back in 1999, one study found that when twenty individuals with CFS removed common food intolerances from their diet, they enjoyed alleviation of their fatigue symptoms.[56] Among the top three dietary intolerances were milk, wheat, and corn. Another trial witnessed significant improvement in physical symptoms and mental outlook in 70 percent of the sixty-four individuals with CFS upon eliminating wheat from their diets.[57] This study also evaluated the use of homeopathic medicines and nutritional supplementation, which present as confounding factors to the research design, making it difficult to understand the effects of wheat-free diet alone. Nevertheless, the dietary aspect should be considered as a vital link as well.

Logan's review article cites two other important studies presented at the American Association for Chronic Fatigue Syndrome conference in 2001.[54] Almost 75 percent of the participants in a Wichita, Kansas group who made dietary modifications reported reduced fatigue. An Australian study found dramatic "improvements in symptom severity across multiple body systems." People with CFS eliminated wheat, milk, and additives such as benzoates, nitrates, and nitrites. An overwhelming 90 percent of these participants experienced significant improvements in fatigue, fever, sore throats, muscle pain, headaches, joint pains, cognitive dysfunction, and irritable bowel-like symptoms. Benefits like these surpass so many of the other treatments and therapies suggested for CFS and yet so little is ever mentioned about natural therapeutic methods like dietary intervention for people with this condition!

Finally, toxin exposures may be related to the food intolerances. Pesticide exposure may inhibit natural tolerance to other chemicals including food products, according to one article. In twenty-two individuals with CFS measured for toxic chemical levels, significantly higher total organochlorine levels were found.[58] Among these organochlorines, more than 90 percent were made up of DDE and hexachlorobenzene. The authors conclude that organically grown fruits and vegetables are important for people with CFS. They also suggest that the CDC definition of CFS should not exclude pesticide exposure since those chemical levels seem elevated in people with CFS. And "bioaccumulation" of low levels of pesticides in the body needs to be further investigated as to its relevance in the disease progression of CFS.

If indeed high levels of toxic chemicals increase the likelihood of developing food intolerances, then perhaps it is not just the foods that cause such symptomatic and inflammatory changes in individuals with CFS. Perhaps the mass use of pesticides in our agriculture has been seeping into our food supply, making certain food groups more symptom-provoking to individuals, leading to chronic illness and conditions such as CFS. Either way, it seems obvious that certain food intolerances worsen symptoms of CFS at the very least. This might be occurring through activation of cytokines, initiating an immune response to those foods. Consequently, eliminating those foods has been shown to be extremely effective in reducing symptoms in the majority of individuals with CFS who were compliant and willing to make such dietary changes.

OXIDATIVE STRESS, MITOCHONDRIAL DYSFUNCTION, AND FREE RADICALS

The fatigue, muscle pain, and other symptoms experienced by those suffering from CFS can be partially attributed to lack of energy produced by cells of the body. When cell structures of the body cannot function properly to create enough energy, the effects show up in the cells, tissues, organs, and of course, the individual as a whole being. One theory behind the chronic fatigue (and also the aging process) is that of oxidative stress created by damage to mitochondria. Mitochondria are cell structures responsible for creating energy for the cell. When they fail to function correctly, they may generate free radicals, compounds that react with and disrupt the integrity of cell components. Free radicals have earned their poor reputation. Not only do they break apart cell membranes and leave the remains of their damage around for the immune system to clean up, they also cause alterations to genes leading toward precancerous cell growth and early aging. Free radicals are also called reactive oxygen species, or oxidants for short. The process by which free radicals produce long-term damage to cells and cell parts is termed oxidative stress.

Antioxidants defend against oxidative stress by binding up free radicals, protecting cells from irreversible damage. It follows that antioxidants not only slow down the aging process but they may also be useful in the treatment of CFS. Emerging research has been focusing on the importance of oxidative stress toward the contribution to CFS, as well as the efficacy of antioxidants to reverse this condition.

Part of this oxidative stress theory was developed by looking at muscle tissue from its physiological and biochemical perspectives. Muscle biopsies taken from volunteers with CFS revealed extensive oxidative damage to the genetic material and lipids (fats) within the specimens collected.[59] Scientists have also found differences in fluidity and fat composition similar to age-related changes in the CFS samples compared to controls. In compensation from this damage to the muscle tissue, the antioxidant enzyme activity had increased. The authors concluded that perhaps CFS has an organic (physiological) cause related to oxidative damage to muscles. In another study, the higher the oxidative stress, the worse the intensity of muscular symptoms for people with CFS.[60] In fact, those with CFS had increased oxidative markers with decreased antioxidant defenses. As recommended by the authors, antioxidant supplementation may relieve the muscle symptoms of pain and tension commonly found in this condition. To confirm these observations, another study found higher blood markers for oxidative stress in people with CFS, which correlated strongly to their symptoms of fatigue, muscle pain, sleep disturbance, and cognitive dysfunction.[61] In fact, even red blood cells can be prone to this oxidative stress, also contributing to the development of CFS.[62] Significant increases in oxidative breakdown products from blood cells, along with increases in antioxidant activity, support the idea of oxidative stress affecting multiple systems in people with CFS. Free radical-induced oxidative stress seems to be a powerful contributor to CFS.

In addition to muscle pain and generalized fatigue, research points to a viable explanation for postexercise fatigue, the feeling of "hitting a wall" with any exertion and being unable to recover even after adequate rest. Oxidative stress to muscles as well as fat tissues can cause this particular symptom of CFS. Oxidation from free radicals can also damage lipids, or fat tissues, including those that make up cholesterol. People with CFS in one study had elevated lipid peroxidation of LDL cholesterol,[63] which contributes toward plaque formation in arteries. These patients also tended to have lower heart-protective cholesterol (HDL) along with the raised oxidized LDL, the latter being the kind that increases rates of heart disease. These changes, along with other blood markers for oxidative stress, were significantly associated with pain and postexercise malaise.[64] Along with those changes, physiological and biochemical testing (for evoked muscle action potential and lactic acid levels) found altered muscle membrane excitability.[59] This kind of muscular dysfunction also explains the muscle pain and postexertional fatigue enhanced from exercise-induced oxidative stress.

Oxidation may be connected to immune system dysfunction in CFS. More recently, a sample of people with CFS revealed significantly higher levels of IgM antibodies against break down products from oxidation such as cell membrane components, products of lipid peroxidation, and amino acid derivatives.[65] Elevated IgM levels correlated with severity of illness from muscle pain and fatigue. The authors speculated that due to oxidative damage, these waste products had become "immunogenic," capable of mounting an immune response. A different research group studied the defective T lymphocyte activation pathways in volunteers with CFS, which correlated to deficiency of zinc in the blood.[66] Inadequate amounts of zinc, accompanied by T cell dysfunction, directly affected symptom severity as well as the "subjective experience of infection" by those afflicted with CFS. This may be another lead into the link between increased oxidative stress of CFS and inadequate amounts of an important antioxidant which also supports the immune system.

An interesting proposal has come forth about one particular oxidant. Peroxynitrite is a powerful oxidant that seems to inactivate mitochondrial enzymes,[67] which have been found to be less active in those with CFS.[68,69] It is thought that a viral infection produces cytokines that enhance the production of peroxynitrite.[67] This oxidant causes mitochondrial dysfunction, lipid peroxidation, and triggers more cytokine release, which only produces more peroxynitrite. It becomes a vicious cycle of peroxynitrite causing increased oxidation leading to further peroxynitrite synthesis. In addition, peroxynitrite lowers activity of the endocrine system, specifically hormones produced by the hypothalamus, pituitary, and adrenal glands. With this influence, glucocorticoids (such as cortisol) are produced in lesser amounts. The next chapter on stress and adrenal gland function explains these concepts in more detail. One scientist comments on peroxynitrite as a common etiology to CFS, multiple chemical sensitivity, and posttraumatic stress disorder.[68] In fact, "peroxynitrite may be the mechanism of a new disease paradigm."

In CFS, as mitochondria become dysfunctional, free radicals or oxidants are generated. These free radicals produce serious damage to multiple organ systems and various tissues of the body, namely the muscles, lipids, cell membranes, and red blood cells. The damage may extend beyond these tissues but these are the ones currently studied in research. Oxidative stress created from this long-term damage correlates with many symptoms of CFS.[70] In fact, muscle pain and exercise fatigue common to people suffering from this condition can be directly attributed to the increased oxidative damage along with reduced antioxidant capacity measured by enzyme activity. Oxidative stress also increases cholesterol peroxidation, which is one of the steps toward atherosclerosis, and increases immune system activity against the products of oxidative damage, which relates to severity of illness. Finally, a particular oxidant (peroxynitrite) may contribute to the slowing down of hormonal glands of the body, reducing release of important substance such as cortisol. Antioxidants, natural chemicals found in many foods, herbs, and in nutraceutical supplements, may prove to be highly efficacious against the damage caused by oxidative stress.

NEUROLOGICAL DISORDERS

Many of the mental difficulties faced by those with CFS can be traced back to organic problems in the brain. Neurological disorders in the brain can lead to symptoms like impaired mental function, dizziness, headaches, anxiety, and depression. Magnetic resonance imaging of the brain shows more abnormal brain scans in people with CFS than in controls (27% compared to 2%).[71] In fact, some scans revealed "small, punctate, subcortical white matter hyperintensities" in the frontal lobe, the area where higher intellectual thought and mental processing take place.[72] These frontal lobe defects may explain some of the more severe cognitive impairment. Brain scan abnormalities, though more common in CFS, did not follow any specific pattern, meaning that not all who had abnormal scans shared the same type of abnormality.[73] Another study found similar numbers of defects between those with CFS and those with clinical depression.[74] Certain measurements of abnormalities were higher in CFS and in AIDS dementia than were in depression, giving support to the hypothesis of viral encephalitis as one cause of CFS.

Another aspect of brain abnormalities, in addition to lesions found on MRI, is that of hypoperfusion, or reduced blood flow to the brain. Even mild reductions of blood flow to the brain can greatly compromise its function. One study found consistently lower perfusion in people with CFS than in healthy volunteers and people with depression.[75] This pattern was especially noticeable in the brainstem, the area of the brain responsible for balance, heart rate, and blood pressure regulation. A similar experiment found diminished blood flow to multiple regions and lobes of the brain, not just the brainstem, in 80 percent of the CFS patients tested.[76] The reduced blood flow occurs in broad areas, and these reductions were more prominent in those who did not experience depression, indicating that this nondepressed group was more likely to have cognitive dysfunction.[77] These two studies provide more pathophysiological evidence for the functional mental impairment experienced by many suffering from CFS.

Reduced blood flow to the brain may be responsible for the dizziness and lack of balance experienced as a common symptom of CFS. In fact, patients tested for their vestibular function performed below average and experienced a significant number of falls.[78] Dysfunction in the central nervous system (primarily the brain) may lead to disequilibrium. Abnormalities in posture while walking represent another indicator of central nervous system (CNS) deficit. Gait abnormalities, as they are commonly referred, are unlikely caused by increasing fatigue with walking.[79] Instead, they are likely manifestations of impairments on the level of the CNS. The higher incidence of gait abnormalities may also have to do with muscle weakness and balance issues in addition to CNS dysfunction.[80]

Symptoms of cognitive dysfunction common to CFS include issues like inability to maintain concentration, slower mental function, headaches, and dizziness, to name just a few. There is evidence of organic problems- abnormal lesions on MRI scans, reduced blood flow to the brain, and cerebral dysfunctions manifesting as disequilibrium. How ironic that so many people with CFS are told that "it's all in your head" when in fact it may really be the case for them!

REVIEW OF ETIOLOGIES

Because CFS has so many roots, it seems silly to try to pigeonhole each individual into just one category. Beyond that, there are overlaps between many of these possible causes so that one etiology may perpetuate another. It would benefit each individual to understand how these issues interplay, and what the role of these etiologies is in the course of the illness.

To summarize, immune dysfunction seems to be a common problem. Instead of deficiency, multiple immune components exhibit "polycellular activation." So treatment approaches should aim to modulate rather than stimulate or suppress the immune system. While no one particular microorganism proves to be the sole cause of CFS, many have been implicated. Infections with EBV and other viruses, Lyme spirochete, and even some bacteria may predispose a person for CFS later on. The persistence of these microbes, as well as higher antibody levels against them, correlates to the severity of illness.

Up to half of those with CFS tend to have history of atopic conditions such as allergies, asthma, and eczema. Many individuals with CFS test positive on RAST tests for environmental and chemical allergies. In addition, many also have symptoms suggestive of food intolerances. Several studies have shown that eliminating dairy, wheat, and corn (common food intolerances) from the diet improves symptoms of CFS.

Table 2.2. Summary of Etiologies and Corresponding Symptoms

Etiology	Abnormalities	Symptoms
Immune system dysfunction	"Polycellular activation": exaggerated responses of T and B lymphocytes, monocytes, natural killer cells, and various chemical factors; low numbers and activity of NK cells	Low-grade fever, swollen lymph nodes, fatigue, malaise, muscle pain, frequent illnesses
Viral and microbial infection	Latent viral infections of EBV, HHV, HLTV, and CMV; bacteria, fungus, spirochetes	Low-grade fever, malaise, swollen lymph nodes, muscle pain, fatigue
Allergies and atopy	Increased eosinophilic cationic proteins, hypersensitivity to environmental, chemical, metal allergens	Interfaces with the neuroendocrine system, leading to fatigue, hormonal, and immune imbalance
Food intolerances	Increased inflammatory cytokines and immune parameters	Fatigue, fever, sore throats, muscle pain, headaches, joint pains, cognitive dysfunction, and irritable bowel-like symptoms
Oxidative stress	Mitochondrial dysfunction, generation of free radicals, disruption of cell membranes including red blood cells, cholesterol peroxidation, activation of immunoglobulins and T lymphocytes, increased peroxynitrites inhibiting hormonal pathways	Fatigue, muscle pain, joint inflammation, aging process, cognitive decline, sleep disturbance, postexercise fatigue
Brain abnormalities	Lesions in various regions and lobes of the brain, cerebral and brainstem hypoperfusion	Cognitive dysfunction, gait abnormalities, dizziness, headaches, loss of balance, anxiety, depression

Increased levels of oxidative stress is common to CFS, affecting multiple organ systems in the body, and leading to symptoms of fatigue, muscle pain, sleep disturbance, and cognitive dysfunction. Mitochondrial dysfunction is the leading cause of free radical production and oxidative damage. And the byproducts of oxidative damage can be "immunogenic" in that they overactivate the immune response, further contributing to illness. And finally, organic lesions of the brain as well as reduced blood flow to the brain may contribute to the cognitive impairment symptoms common to CFS. Table 2.2 summarizes each of these potential causes along with the associated abnormalities and symptoms.

CHAPTER 3

Stress, Adrenal Fatigue, and Cognitive Disorder

Stress seems to be an everyday part of life nowadays, and this word has become common parlance to describe all means of difficulty and adversity. Many believe that being in physical pain due to illness is stressful. Or that being exposed to the multitudes of chemicals in our environment wears us down. Even dealing with uncomfortable life situations and being around provoking people can be extremely stressful for most. No matter the source of stress, though, the human body has a predictable pattern of responding to it. This stress response was first described in the 1930s by Dr. Hans Selye as the general adaptation syndrome. Since that time, much medical research continues to elaborate on the complexities of this mechanism used by the body to compensate for the onslaught of stressful experiences endured. While there is a predictable sequence of physical and chemical reactions in the body for most people, some of these reactions may be altered or abnormal or extreme. In the study of chronic fatigue syndrome (CFS), we find that the typical stress response has been affected. It largely resembles that of adrenal fatigue or vital exhaustion, commonly referred to colloquially as "burnout." Stress is probably one of the most important factors to evaluate when figuring out why an individual has CFS.

THE HYPOTHALAMUS-PITUITARY-ADRENAL AXIS

Many experts on CFS believe this condition to be one of a neuroendocrine imbalance rather than an immunological dysfunction. This means that CFS affects people at the level of the brain and its connections with hormonal systems in the body. This theory of nervous and hormonal dysregulation ties together the diverse issues of stress, long-term fatigue, sleep disturbances, and immune system dysfunction. In fact, people with less than optimal function of the adrenal gland, a condition known as hypoadrenalism or adrenal insufficiency, also show symptoms of fatigue, muscle weakness, lightheadedness, cognitive disorders, allergies, and weakened immune response very similar to those seen in CFS. In both conditions, there may be dysregulation of the adrenal gland function.

First, let us review the impact of stress on the adrenal gland's production of hormones. The adrenal gland serves as the body's survival organ. It provides resilience in the face of stress and adversity. A healthy stress response involves secretion of hormones such as epinephrine, norepinephrine, cortisol, and many others. Both epinephrine and norepinephrine have stimulating effects on the body; they quicken breathing rate and heart rate, increase blood pressure, enhance cardiac output of oxygen-rich blood to nourish the rest of the body, improve direct blood flow to the skeletal muscles in anticipation of activity, and increase rate of metabolism overall. These effects, known as the sympathetic "fight or flight" response, provide the energy needed to confront or escape a dangerous situation. In prehistoric times, adrenal hormones epinephrine and norepinephrine gave humans the gusto to hunt wild animals and the speed to run away from the proverbial saber-toothed tiger if the hunt was unsuccessful. In present times, even as the reality of hunting and fleeing have faded into the past, the human body still responds in the same way physiologically to mental and emotional stressors. This phenomenon partially explains the high blood pressure, panic and anxiety, shallow breathing, and fast irregular pulse that arise during times of high stress.

In addition to epinephrine and norepinephrine, the adrenal gland releases other hormones to affect the stress response in the long-term. The cortex, or outer shell, of the adrenal gland secretes glucocorticoids (such as cortisol), mineralocorticoids, and steroids (such as androgens and DHEA). Androgens include the sex hormones testosterone and its hormonal precursors that exhibit masculinizing effects: facial hair, denser bones, bulkier muscles, and so on. DHEA, which stands for dehydroepiandrosterone, is an androgen hormone that converts into the sex hormones testosterone and estrogen. Mineralocorticoids keep electrolytes (minerals like sodium and potassium) in balance with one another in the bloodstream to regulate blood volume and blood pressure. Glucocorticoids deliver nutrients through the bloodstream to feed the different cells and tissues and organs of the body in times of stress.

Cortisol, a classic glucocorticoid, has the overall effect of breaking down stored fats and proteins and carbohydrates to make these nutrients available for use as energy in the body. Cortisol output is tightly regulated by a hormone made by the pituitary gland in the brain called adrenocorticotropic hormone (ACTH). ACTH prods the adrenal gland to make more cortisol and release it into the bloodstream so that the different organs and tissues of the body can be nourished with energy sources. At other times, ACTH can also respond to high levels of cortisol by telling the adrenal gland to slow down its productivity. Consequently, the pituitary gland, through output of ACTH, controls how much cortisol gets made and released by the adrenal gland to influence the levels of nutrients in the bloodstream. Cortisol release exhibits certain unique patterns throughout the day (and night). The highest amount is released in the early morning upon awakening, and then the levels gradually fade throughout the rest of the day until they reach a minimal point at night. These unique patterns are termed diurnal rhythms when they occur during the daytime and during periods of light, or circadian rhythms when they are assessed during a 24-hour cycle.

During periods of high stress, ACTH stimulates higher cortisol production to break down stored compounds into energy sources for the body. After chronic or prolonged periods of stress, negative consequences start to occur from chronically elevated levels of glucocorticoids. High circulating fat levels deposit into blood vessels predisposing the individual to cardiovascular disease. High levels of glucose in the bloodstream may deposit into organs provoking early consequences of type II diabetes mellitus. Changes in blood glucose levels also affect the way the body responds to insulin, leading to insulin resistance, creating a vicious cycle of fat deposition into adipose tissue, ultimately increasing central adiposity or "belly fat." Meanwhile, excessive protein breakdown can reduce much needed muscle mass into fats and carbohydrates. This in turn lowers the resting metabolic rate causing easy fatigue, muscle weakness, and reduced endurance.

On the other hand, dysfunction of the autonomic nervous system, which is responsible for our stress response, can cause shutting down of the adrenal glands. As adrenal gland function slows down, cortisol output declines. Insufficient production of cortisol can have effects such as hypoglycemia (low blood glucose levels), fatigue, weakness, muscle pain, anxiety, depression, and loss of mental acuity. People with this condition may experience generalized weakness and malaise, lack of energy, cognitive difficulties, low blood pressure, poor immune function, and tendency toward becoming lightheaded due to low blood sugar levels. These symptoms of adrenal burnout may also be experienced by people with CFS.

All of the effects of the adrenal glands depend on proper working of the hypothalamus, an area of the brain that commands the pituitary gland to stimulate other glands of the body. The hypothalamus releases various hormones to cause the pituitary gland to release its own myriad of hormones in turn. These pituitary hormones boost endocrine glands all throughout the body to make their own respective hormones. In the case of the adrenals, the hypothalamus secretes corticotrophin releasing hormone (CRH) to push the pituitary to secrete more ACTH. This enhances production of cortisol by the adrenals. Normally, higher cortisol levels will feedback to the hypothalamus and the pituitary to slow down release of their respective hormones. In this way, overall cortisol production is kept in check. However, once the adrenal glands reach a level of "burn out," it takes increasing secretions of CRH and ACTH to jumpstart the adrenals. At this point, no matter how much CRH and ACTH are released, the adrenal glands can only secrete insufficient amounts of cortisol. This becomes a condition known as adrenal insufficiency.

Going back to CFS, the effects of cortisol and ACTH can explain various aspects of CFS symptoms. Indeed, activation of the stress system leads to changes that improve an individual's chances for survival. However, long-term activation of the stress system leads to negative consequences at the hypothalamic-pituitary-adrenal gland connection, mimicking adrenal insufficiency in the end.

The adrenal glands may at first heighten their response to ACTH by producing more cortisol, and later shut down by making less. Also, the pituitary gland may become less responsive to hypothalamic prodding, becoming less able to produce ACTH. Either way, these chronic changes perpetuate the symptoms of fatigue, sleep disorders, cognitive issues, muscle pains, and immune system dysfunctions seen in people with CFS. As so many of these symptoms of CFS and adrenal gland dysfunction overlap, research has been focused on finding the links between these two conditions to understand the development of chronic fatigue.

CORTISOL AND ITS ROLE IN CFS

Since its first suggestion in the 1950s, the theory of adrenal insufficiency correlating with CFS has been gaining popularity.[1] More and more research studies are focusing on reduced hypothalamic-pituitary-adrenal activity as part of the pathology of CFS. Many experts have proposed cortisol as a primary link between adrenal insufficiency and CFS. In fact, people with CFS tend to have lower cortisol levels in general, pointing to limited adrenal functioning as an important mechanism for this condition.

Several studies have proposed reduced cortisol production in people with CFS. In one of these studies, people with CFS had overall reduced cortisol response.[2] Monitoring their urinary cortisol levels for 24 hours found significantly reduced overall excretion which meant significantly less cortisol production. In addition, lower evening cortisol levels with higher evening ACTH levels pointed to an abnormal adrenal response to the pituitary stimulus. The authors suggest a lowered ACTH response to CRH and an increased sensitivity of the adrenals to ACTH. So, the adrenal insufficiency seen in people with CFS may be due to insufficient production of CRH in the hypothalamus.

In another study, people with CFS showed a significantly lower cortisol output when given CRH to stimulate the pituitary gland's release of ACTH, and fenfluramine to stimulate the hypothalamus to secrete releasing hormones.[3] This meant that the adrenal glands were responding poorly to both CRH and ACTH. When this same group was given hydrocortisone to stimulate the adrenal glands, they showed significantly higher cortisol production in response to CRH. In this case, the lower cortisol levels may be due to less than optimal function of the adrenal glands.

People with CFS whose urine was measured for cortisol every 3 hours between 6 A.M. and 9 P.M. showed a normal diurnal rhythm.[4] Again, diurnal, or circadian, rhythms are unique cycles of biological activity that occur at about the same time everyday. So in this case, people with CFS exhibited normal patterns for releasing varying amounts of cortisol throughout the day. However, these individuals showed lower levels of cortisol throughout the day's measurements compared to the healthy control group. In another study, people with CFS were assessed over 2 days for their awakening and circadian cortisol levels.[5] They showed normal circadian rhythms. However, after receiving injections of dexamethasone, a pharmaceutical drug to feedback to the pituitary gland to slow down secretion of ACTH, they exhibited prolonged suppression of cortisol production compared to the control group. To summarize, these two studies confirm with one another that the circadian rhythms of cortisol release may be normal in people with CFS. Yet, they seem to produce smaller quantities of cortisol overall. And when the pituitary gland is held back from stimulating the adrenal glands, there is an abnormally longer suppression of cortisol synthesis. Perhaps people with CFS have slower adrenal response to ACTH, again supporting the idea of reduced cortisol from adrenal-pituitary dysfunction.

Aside from 24-hour urinary collections, other studies have started measuring cortisol levels in the saliva of people with CFS. This salivary collection technique enables researchers to assess levels every few hours and to witness more accurate patterns as opposed to a total single collection at the end. For example, one study found no difference in the activity of the hypothalamus-pituitary-adrenal axis with a single 24-hour collection of both urinary and salivary cortisol in people with CFS compared to healthy controls.[6] Perhaps using various measurements throughout this time period would have produced more specific results. Case in point, the authors of one study call salivary cortisol collection a more "naturalistic measure of HPA function" in that it is less invasive and more informative than other techniques. They discovered that morning salivary cortisol levels upon awakening were consistently lower among people with CFS.[7] In a previously mentioned study, a group of researchers measured salivary cortisol every 3 hours from 6 A.M. to 9 P.M. and found similar results to urinary cortisol levels assessed in the same way.[8] Both studies confirmed that cortisol levels, as well as its precursor cortisone, were significantly lower over the whole day, with the only exception being at 9 P.M. And, as in other cases, diurnal rhythms were similar to controls. The majority of the evidence reinforces the theory that HPA dysfunction negatively affects the adrenal glands' ability to make cortisol in people with CFS.

A thought arose among researchers as to whether giving cortisol to people with CFS would actually improve their natural ability to make more cortisol. People taking oral hydrocortisone (pharmaceutical cortisol) for 3 months showed improvement in their Wellness scores on more days than untreated people.[9] However, the authors of this study found enough adverse effects due to adrenal suppression which in their minds precluded the practical usage of this medication to curb the symptoms of CFS. Since then, other studies testing the symptomatic and physiological benefits of similar drugs have failed to show significant improvements. Fludrocortisone (in the same category as hydrocortisone) did not offer any advantages to symptoms, blood pressure, heart rate, and other biochemical factors.[10] And Synacthen, another corticosteroid, given to people with CFS showed no difference in cortisol responses compared to controls.[11] Authors of these studies propose that insufficient production of cortisol alone may not fully explain the process of CFS, and that other factors such as poor sleep, inactivity, circadian disruptors, chronic illness, medications, and psychiatric disorders need to be addressed.

Finally, some have suggested a link between clinical burnout, vital exhaustion, and CFS because of overlap between symptoms. However, CFS stands apart from other stress-related conditions. One research study found no difference in people with clinical burnout regarding the awakening cortisol levels and HPA feedback with dexamethasone.[12] In both clinical burnout and CFS the dexamethasone suppression test caused prolonged cortisol suppression as well in people with chronic fatigue. Yet in another study, people with burnout had higher cortisol levels upon awakening and up to 1 hour afterward.[13] With burnout, dysregulation of HPA activity is experienced through elevated levels of morning cortisol, whereas people with CFS exhibit lower morning cortisol levels. In another similar condition called vital exhaustion (characterized by extreme fatigue, irritability, and demoralization), a lower basal cortisol production occurs in the evening, as opposed to morning in CFS.[14] These lower evening cortisol levels in vital exhaustion can be explained by chronic stress leading to sleep disturbance and end-of-day fatigue.

To summarize, CFS exhibits lower overall cortisol levels, lower morning cortisol levels, and generally normal diurnal rhythms. In addition, people with CFS produce less cortisol overall partially due to less than optimal functioning of their adrenal glands (like in adrenal insufficiency) and also due to change in responsiveness to ACTH and CRH. Insufficient cortisol response in CFS can be attributed to adrenal gland dysfunction as well as problems at the level of the hypothalamus and pituitary glands.

HYPOTHALAMUS AND PITUITARY DYSFUNCTION IN CFS

Reduced cortisol synthesis in CFS has been blamed on two main factors: reduced function of the adrenal glands, and changes in the secretions of ACTH from the pituitary as well as CRH from the hypothalamus. In fact "HPA" stands for hypothalamus-pituitary-adrenal, and this three-gland axis upholds and vetoes one another according to situation. The hypothalamus and pituitary, glands that sit within the brain, are just as responsible for the hormonal dysfunction of CFS as are the adrenal glands. There is some early evidence to explain how this happens.

It is believed that CFS is exacerbated by physical as well as mental and emotional stressors. Research upholds the idea that these stressors lead to HPA dysfunction causing hormonal imbalances.[15] As a general rule, people with CFS have reduced HPA activity due to "impaired CNS drive," according to a couple of experts who have studied the unique characteristics of this system. The impairment involves both the hypothalamus and the pituitary glands. Interestingly, this HPA impairment is different from what is observed in people with depression or other mental-emotional disorders. The evidence for impaired activity goes back to the early 1990s when a study showed overall "blunted" or insufficient ACTH response to the hypothalamus secreting CRH.[16] People with CFS were given artificial CRH to test the pituitary and adrenal responses to this hormone by measuring urinary cortisol output. The pituitary gland released less ACTH despite being provoked by artificial CRH, revealing a blunted response. In compensation, the adrenal glands seemed more sensitive to ACTH, even if still not producing enough cortisol. Oddly, evening pituitary secretions of ACTH were actually elevated, suggesting that the issue is not entirely about the pituitary gland.

The authors concluded that CFS is not a condition of the adrenal glands but one of deficiency of CRH or other hormones that stimulate the pituitary-adrenal pathway.

Several other studies support this theory.[17,18,19,20] In a more recent trial, people with CFS given artificial CRH had significantly reduced ACTH release and reduced cortisol production.[17] Perhaps, as these experts propose, there may be abnormal CRH levels or altered pituitary sensitivity to CRH. Or the dysregulation has to do with other hormones influencing the HPA axis. Vasopressin is one such influential pituitary hormone which will be discussed later.

But what if dysregulation of HPA hormones is a consequence of the condition rather than a cause? Blood samples were assayed for various hormones every hour for a full 24-hour cycle in a group of fifteen medication-free individuals with CFS.[18] Not surprisingly, morning ACTH levels, between 8 A.M. and 10 A.M., were much lower in people with CFS compared to healthy volunteers. And the overall ACTH rhythm or circadian pattern was also lower. No significant differences were found in cortisol or other pituitary hormones such as growth hormone (GH) and prolactin. Because of this discrepancy of lower ACTH but normal cortisol levels, the authors wonder if these changes are more likely a result instead of an etiology of CFS.

A battery of different tests was given to both healthy volunteers and people with CFS to compare hormone responses.[19] To ascertain both physical and mental-emotional reactions to stress, this study used a psychological stress test and a standardized exercise test in response to a procedure mimicking a real-life stressor. All three tests showed reduced ACTH responses in people with CFS. However, cortisol response was higher in reaction to the insulin tolerance test but not the stress and exercise tests. In other words, people with CFS can mount sufficient cortisol responses during stress, but not ACTH responses. Instead, ACTH levels actually go down as a result of stress. This again points to subtle alterations at the hypothalamus-pituitary level.

People with CFS evaluated for neuroendocrine function using the insulin tolerance test showed significantly reduced ACTH response in another study as well.[20] And this ACTH reduction was significantly associated with the duration of CFS symptoms as well as the severity of fatigue. This study reinforces the relation between HPA alterations and symptoms of CFS. Although there is still some confusion about why this relation exists, one theory lies in the behavior patterns of many people who suffer from CFS. The perpetuating factors for the chronic nature of CFS, like profound inactivity, deconditioning of physical fitness, and abnormal sleep patterns, may be leading up to some of this neuroendocrine imbalance. Again the chicken versus egg question comes up of whether this imbalance is a risk factor for CFS, or whether CFS in fact produces this imbalance. If the latter has some validity, it may serve as a way to measure prognosis, or the likelihood that the individual with CFS will improve or worsen.

Stress negatively influences the hypothalamus-pituitary-adrenal axis, reducing the ability of these organs to secrete proper amounts of hormones. Not only do the adrenal glands produce less cortisol in CFS, the pituitary gland also fails to secrete enough ACTH. These alterations of the HPA axis suggest an influence higher up. Either the hypothalamic secretions of CRH do not suffice, or other pituitary hormones may be getting in the way. Or perhaps all of these hormonal imbalances stem from the condition itself along with its perpetuating behavioral factors. In the latter case, unfortunately, people with CFS may be perpetuating their CFS symptoms and HPA dysfunction by poorly dealing with their level of suffering. Nevertheless, the reduced ACTH is directly associated with CFS symptoms and severity of fatigue. And these clues about ACTH (and other HPA alterations) must be further studied to reveal connections with the etiology and the consequences of CFS.

HORMONES THAT INFLUENCE THE HPA AXIS

Many hormones influence the HPA axis, aside from cortisol, ACTH, and CRH. Candidates include DHEA, vasopressin, and perhaps even melatonin, growth hormone, and insulin-like growth factor (IGF). Several studies have tried to understand the relationship between these hormones and the imbalances present that exacerbate CFS symptoms.

One such hormone, DHEA, is an adrenal hormone that converts into sex hormones such as estrogen, progesterone, and testosterone. This hormone is said to contribute to other physiologic factors such as memory, depression, sleep, weight loss, and even longevity. It is often called the "miracle hormone" because of its role in counteracting the negative effects of cortisol and stress. In a preliminary study,[19] chronically fatigued individuals given ACTH exhibited higher DHEA levels compared to the control group.[21] In these individuals, the ACTH seemed to stimulate more DHEA production rather than cortisol. Those with CFS did not exhibit the reduced proportion of DHEA compared to cortisol in response to ACTH the way that the control group did. The authors think that this inappropriate stress response with elevated DHEA and insufficient cortisol is common in CFS.

Another study found that baseline levels of DHEA were higher in those with CFS.[22] And this elevation in DHEA correlated with increased disability scores. Those with CFS who were treated with hydrocortisone exhibited lower DHEA levels than those who were not treated. After being given CRH to stimulate adrenal hormone production, individuals with CFS had a small (statistically insignificant) rise in DHEA. But those whose fatigue improved from treatment with hydrocortisone showed increased DHEA response to CRH. And so, the hydrocortisone therapy reduces baseline DHEA levels to normal but also improves the adrenal output of DHEA from CRH influence. It seems that people with CFS tend to have lower cortisol levels with elevated DHEA levels, both of which correspond to disability. The higher DHEA levels can be normalized by treatment with hydrocortisone, which reduces these levels while improving the adrenal response to CRH.

One of the signs of autonomic nervous system dysfunction from chronic stress is lowered blood pressure with light-headedness from standing up too quickly.

This symptom is common in CFS and serves as a tool for understanding the HPA imbalance. The main hormone responsible for maintaining blood pressure upon standing up from a seated position is vasopressin, also known as antidiuretic hormone. Vasopressin is a pituitary hormone with an adrenal influence. It prevents dehydration, retains water within the body, sustains adequate blood pressure, and prevents lightheadedness. It also plays a role in stimulating ACTH release by the pituitary gland, as well as indirectly stimulating the adrenal glands to produce their respective hormones. When the pituitary and adrenal glands fail to respond properly to vasopressin, the resulting dehydration and low cortisol output reduce blood pressure. This may lead to orthostatic hypotension or neural-mediated hypotension, the symptoms of lowered blood pressure and lightheadedness upon suddenly standing up.

Vasopressin has been used to evaluate the influence CRH has on the pituitary gland. In fact, some experts believe that vasopressin works synergistically with CRH to enhance the pituitary gland's ACTH secretions. One study used a synthetic form of vasopressin to augment this ACTH response in individuals with CFS.[23] The CFS group already showed lowered ACTH and cortisol responses to stimulation by CRH. Administering vasopressin did not cause a significant difference in these responses between the CFS group and the control group. However, when given both vasopressin and CRH together, the chronic fatigue individuals showed significantly increased cortisol output. The ACTH levels also rose, but slightly, in this same group. This suggests that vasopressin improves the pituitary response to CRH only in individuals with CFS. And that maybe vasopressin exerts its influence on both the pituitary gland's production of ACTH, as well as the adrenal glands' production of cortisol.

Another study that infused people with CFS with vasopressin showed a slightly different response.[24] The CFS group experienced lowered ACTH responses in this case. However, their cortisol responses were much more rapid as a result. A possible explanation is that vasopressin activated the HPA axis in some way as to stimulate the already low CRH secretion from the hypothalamus.

Growth hormone, or GH, which is also secreted from the pituitary gland, has been shown to be related to conditions related to CFS. In fibromyalgia, for example, the presence of GH has been found to be very low. This deficit of GH might be what spurs on sleep and neuroendocrine disturbances specific to fibromyalgia.[25] In general, the role of GH is to stimulate growth of bones, tissues, and organs of the body. GH enhances protein synthesis, uses up fat stores, and conserves carbohydrates. It also signals the release of insulin-like growth factor (IGF) which further enhances the effect of GH on the development of body tissues. Both GH and IGF levels appear to be lower in people suffering from fibromyalgia, and it has been postulated that this may also be true for people with CFS.

However, several research studies suggest lack of significant differences in GH and IGF in people with CFS compared to controls.[25,26,27] Baseline IGF levels were similar in both groups, and there were no differences in the GH responses to stimulatory tests in either group.[26] Some conclude that the GH-IGF axis is not impaired in CFS the way it is in fibromyalgia.[27]

Another study evaluated levels of GH and IGF in individuals with CFS, along with confirming known cortisol, ACTH, and other hormonal imbalances.[28] In contrast to the previously mentioned studies, the CFS volunteers in this one showed significantly decreased GH response to induced hypoglycemia. Normally, hypoglycemia stimulates a rise in the secretion of GH. Also, nocturnal GH secretion was impaired, where normally it should be higher at night than during the day. Oddly, these changes in GH did not lead to any significant fluctuations in IGF concentrations. And this more recent study conflicts with past literature. So, it becomes difficult to determine the role of GH and IGF in the perpetuation of CFS.

Melatonin is another such controversial hormone. It is released by the pineal gland deep in the brain to synchronize circadian rhythms of night and day cycles in the body. Melatonin allows for restful deep sleep and adequate energy. While melatonin levels tend to be higher at night in people with fibromyalgia, there is no significant difference in the levels in women with CFS compared to controls.[29] Also, there seems to be no change in the timing of melatonin and cortisol secretory patterns between the two groups. Melatonin might be a valuable tool for gauging the susceptibility for HPA disruptions from stress. But so far, it does not offer much connection with CFS.

Some research has tried to assess whether chemicals similar to hormones play a role in CFS development. Neurotransmitters are important chemicals thought to influence not just the brain but also many other organs of the body. Some of these neurotransmitters strongly affect moods and behaviors, influencing depression, panic, anxiety, euphoria, and pain perception to name just a few. One study found significant changes in levels of neurotransmitter metabolites in people with CFS.[30] These breakdown substances are compatible with symptoms of "chronic lethargy and fatigue with persistent immune stimulation." These metabolites may turn out to be specific biological markers for diagnosing the severity of this condition. Other research refutes this idea of a difference in neurotransmitters in CFS. One study showed no difference in the serotonin levels and depression scores in people with CFS compared to controls.[31] Perhaps serotonin may not play an important role in the development of this condition. Another study found no association between opioid levels and the secretions of ACTH and cortisol.[32] Opioids, natural pain-relieving substances found in the brain and elsewhere in the body, were once thought to influence the HPA activity of people with CFS.

SUMMARY OF HPA AXIS AND HORMONES

While neurotransmitters may or may not play an important part in the development of CFS, it seems that many hormones do. The pituitary gland's secretion of ACTH causes a rise in the DHEA output from the adrenal glands, without a relative increase in cortisol production. Also, treatment with synthetic cortisol (hydrocortisone) reduces DHEA and its corresponding symptoms of disability, while improving the adrenal responses to ACTH. These imbalanced proportions of ACTH, cortisol, and DHEA suggest an inappropriate stress response in people with CFS. Vasopressin works hand-in-hand with CRH from the hypothalamus to activate the pituitary gland. This hormone supports the adrenal production of cortisol via the HPA axis. Additionally, there appear to be few commonalities to fibromyalgia in terms of changes in growth hormone, IGF, and melatonin levels. Most research shows little difference in these hormones for people with CFS compared to nonfatigued individuals. Only one study suggests depressed GH responses to hypoglycemia and lower night time GH secretion in CFS. There is still much to uncover about the connection between GH-IGF axis and the HPA axis.

Overall, many who suffer from CFS do so in part because of lowered cortisol levels. The adrenal glands may not be responding to higher hormonal influences. They may be slowing down after chronic stress activation just like in adrenal insufficiency or "burnout." Occasionally, higher evening or nighttime cortisol levels may be observed, causing sleep disturbances at night. This situation compounded with lower morning levels of cortisol, when it should be peaking, explains the sluggishness and lethargy experienced by many individuals with CFS. Often times, the adrenal glands can in fact produce sufficient quantities of cortisol at normal circadian rhythms. However, the ACTH hormone that activates cortisol production by the adrenals is too low. ACTH is a hormone released by the pituitary gland in the brain in response to CRH from the hypothalamus. In many CFS individuals, this ACTH release is "blunted" or reduced despite CRH stimulation. In compensation, the adrenal glands may actually become more sensitive to ACTH since there is very little of this hormone. Interestingly, ACTH output actually goes down in response to physical, mental, or emotional stress. Whether the reduced ACTH increases susceptibility to CFS or whether CFS induces blunted ACTH responses is not yet clear. Either way, stress exerts many negative consequences on the HPA axis and upon the development and perpetuation of CFS. And therapy needs to be focused on nourishing both the adrenal glands, as well as supporting the hormonal axis with its response to stress.

WHAT'S STRESS GOT TO DO WITH IT?

Beyond all the intricate details and complexities of the hormonal systems of the body lies the underlying culprit—stress. No one is immune to stress, however everyone has her own unique reaction to life's difficulties. Some of life's hardships and crises wear down on us physically. The signs and symptoms are pretty obvious: tense shoulders, frequent headaches, insomnia, sugar cravings, addiction to caffeine and other stimulants, dependency on alcohol for tension relief, poor immune resilience, depression, and of course, fatigue. Stress exerts its negative influences on the body via disrupting the HPA axis. It can also wreak havoc within the rest of the neuroendocrine system, as well as the immune system and cardiovascular system. The effects can be witnessed as part of many various health conditions, and CFS is no exception.

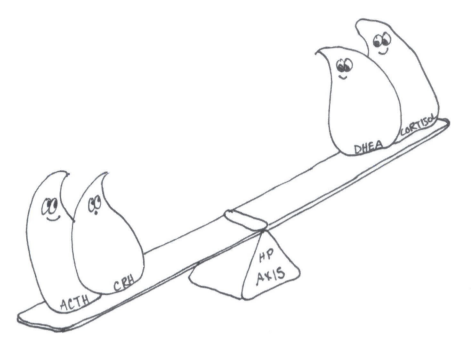

Figure 3.1. The HPA axis is a delicate balance of hormoncs ACTH, CRH, DHEA, cortisol. *Courtesy of Taunya Jernigan.*

Life's emotional distresses seem to provoke the onset of CFS. In one report, individuals with CFS were more likely to experience severe events or difficulties within 3 months to 1 year prior to the onset of their condition.[33] While no one from the control group suffered distress, 30 percent of the CFS group dealt with a major stressful event only 3 months before developing their chronic fatigue. Emotional stress is obviously one of several causative factors for CFS and it is a very likely contributor indeed.

To evaluate the effects of critical life events on chronic fatigue, CFS volunteers were asked to identify life events, the month prior to illness when they occurred, and the symptoms and intensity during that time.[34] Three months prior to developing CFS, individuals reached much higher fatigue, pain, and fever levels versus the control group. These levels stayed higher throughout the entire first year of illness while those in the control group experienced a rapid decline in their levels. The prevalence of negative life events to occur 3 months prior doubled in the CFS group compared to control. The prevalence of infections successively increased in the 3 months prior to onset for the CFS group and not the control.

In other words, the CFS individuals had clues about the onset of their condition a few months to a year prior to the actual beginning. And these symptomatic clues were related to the doubled rate of negative life events in the CFS group. Perhaps individuals with CFS have a reduced tolerance for and impaired ability to withstand high levels of emotional distress found in certain difficult life events.

Understanding stress sensitivity will help health-care providers create a therapy that includes this unique mind-body component of CFS.

COGNITIVE DYSFUNCTION

CFS is characterized by its ability to affect mental functioning. This cognitive impairment manifests with symptoms such as learning difficulties, inability to maintain concentration, slower information processing speed, memory loss, and others. These issues profoundly impact the quality of life for many individuals, and they do not seem related to psychological illness such as depression. Instead, these mental symptoms are specific and unique to CFS.

When given tests on memory, attention, and information processing, individuals with CFS scored poorly compared to controls, with no relation to severity of psychiatric illness.[35] This means that whether or not these individuals also suffered from depression, they still failed to perform adequately on cognitive tests. In a study comparing cognitive functioning among patients with CFS, depression, and multiple sclerosis, the CFS group showed the most significant impairment in information processing among the three groups.[36] Their level of depression and anxiety did not seem to make a difference in their scores. Significant differences in learning and memory remained regardless of severity of psychiatric illness and despite using or discontinuing use of psychiatric medications.[37] Even among CFS patients who did not exhibit depression, many showed a generally "lower positive affect," or lower overall mood, associated with slower cognitive processing and motor speed.[38]

In a study of forty-three individuals with CFS, those with significant complaints of mental fatigue showed greater impairment in tasks requiring memory and sustained attention.[39] While they started out normally, these individuals seemed to experience increasing mental fatigue as the testing process continued. In other words, their subjective experience of mental fatigue correlated directly with cognitive impairment observed in testing. In fact, individuals with CFS tend to be similar to those with multiple sclerosis in that they both have difficulty with simultaneous processing of complex cognitive information.[40] In addition, they seem to have difficulties with attention as well as a "reduced information processing speed and efficiency."[41] This reduced attention span hinders their ability to conduct tasks requiring planning and responding based on memory.[42] One researcher commented on the effects of this cognitive impairment in quality of life in that "everyday cognitive tasks may require excessive processing resources leaving patients with diminished spare attentional capacity or flexibility."[43]

This brings to mind the issue of reduced blood flow to the brain—perhaps this organic problem manifests symptomatically as inefficient information processing. A larger study of 141 CFS patients found that they were more likely than controls to fail at least one test of attention, speed of information processing, or motor speed (but not on measures of memory and executive functioning).[44] They consistently scored lower on reaction-time tasks where cognitive and motor speeds were critical.[45] And they underperformed on a greater variety of cognitive tests across the board.

While there is no clear explanation of why individuals with CFS tend to have cognitive disorders, there is one interesting finding. There may exist a genetic factor involved in the cognitive impairment of CFS. Monozygotic twins performed worse on speed-dependent tests than healthy twins.[46] They seemed to share a genetic trait related to information processing issues in this condition. Future research will reveal if a genetic test would act as a diagnostic marker for CFS.

DEPRESSION

Depression seems a likely consequence from developing CFS. It seems reasonable that a person dealing with symptoms of CFS with impaired quality of life would be feeling depressed. However, the two conditions, depression and CFS, tend to overlap and many individuals start out having psychiatric illness even before developing chronic fatigue.

Individuals with CFS were more likely to also suffer from depression compared to controls with just fatigue.[47] Not only did they have preexisting psychiatric disorders, but they also had concurrent psychiatric disorders and mood disorders. Depression is more prevalent in CFS as well as its related condition fibromyalgia.[48] This higher prevalence of unrecognized current depression often predated that of the chronic fatigue. Several studies support this finding.[49,50,51] In fact, those with CFS tend to be at a higher risk for concurrent psychiatric disorder than those who do not suffer from chronic fatigue.[52] Up to 75 percent of individuals with CFS may at some time experience a psychiatric illness simultaneously and are more likely to receive psychotropic medication if not already using one.

Psychiatric illness can have detrimental consequences to other systems in the body. Unfortunately, depression does not support the immune system. Patients with CFS who concurrently also had psychiatric illness recovered more slowly to infection with influenza virus. Depression also has an effect on the neuroendocrine system—it reduces synthesis of cortisol. Individuals with CFS and fibromyalgia tend to experience abnormally low levels of cortisol in the morning, further contributing to their symptomatology.[53] Exactly why depression and CFS are correlated still remains unanswered, but there is evidence to support the way that depression comes on even before the onset of CFS and the ways that depression seems to negatively affect both the immune system function as well as endocrine function of the adrenal gland.

PART II

How Is Chronic Fatigue Syndrome Diagnosed?

CHAPTER 4

Standard Diagnosis

So far, no single diagnostic test confirms whether or not a person has chronic fatigue syndrome (CFS). This is part of the difficulty in correct diagnosis. Diagnosis is often based on the physician's ability to ascertain if the person's symptoms match the defining criteria set out by the Centers for Disease Control and Prevention (CDC).[1] Even when they do fit the criteria, other conditions causing fatigue need to be ruled out first before determining that the individual has CFS. There are, in fact, multitudes of conditions that induce chronic fatigue as one of the main symptoms. Fatigue is considered to be one of the most common complaints of individuals seeking medical attention. So the dilemma is to isolate true CFS out of the many disorders leading to generalized fatigue.

Laboratory testing in an individual presenting with chronic fatigue serves two purposes: to rule out other conditions explaining the patient's symptoms, and to recognize diseases that may occur concomitantly or simultaneously to affect overall health. It is easy to overlook the fact that a person may suffer from more than one condition at a time. For example, an individual already suffering from one condition that presents with fatigue could suddenly develop characteristic symptoms that match the CFS criteria. Overlapping symptoms and disorders are common and specific studies may be required to evaluate them. One of the most difficult responsibilities for the physician is to figure out where the fatigue is coming from, and whether or not the individual has CFS. Once this deductive work is accomplished, treatment can be directed at removing the root of the problem and offering therapeutic support for the person's healing process to begin.

Many conditions manifest with symptoms similar to CFS. These include a variety of autoimmune diseases, blood disorders, thyroid and adrenal disease, and other endocrine disorders such as panhypopituitarism, diabetes, and ovarian failure. In addition, some gastrointestinal disorders such as irritable bowel syn-drome and inflammatory bowel disease can also present like CFS. Multiple viral, bacterial, fungal, and parasitic infections, as well as immune disorders, share the same ailments of fatigue and malaise and swollen lymph nodes as CFS. Psychiatric illness such as anxiety, depression, bipolar, sleep disorders, and even muscular dys-trophy can manifest with severe fatigue. Some diseases are considered overlapping illnesses with CFS. These include, but are not limited to, fibromyalgia, Gulf War Syndrome, and multiple chemical sensitivities or environmental illness.[1] The list is quite comprehensive, and it would be unrealistic to try to evaluate for each one with laboratory tests.

Instead, the most useful and cost-effective laboratory tests that are pretty standard to primary care medicine can be used to exclude many other illnesses. These tests can be easily performed from a single blood draw at the order or request of most primary care physicians. Until more research comes through with evidence of better diagnostic procedures, CFS will remain a condition of exclusion. But at least with the following tests, most other conditions can be eliminated, and then the ultimate diagnosis can rest on the CDC criteria.

RECOMMENDED STANDARD LABORATORY TESTS

Complete Blood Count

A complete blood count, or CBC, is the measure of the number of red blood cells, white blood cells, platelets (blood clotting cell fragments), and a differential count of each type of white blood cell. A CBC test is very commonly performed on most people when they go for an annual physical checkup because it provides good information about the quality of the blood. This test can rule out anemia, which commonly presents with fatigue, and viral infections and certain types of cancers, which may cause abnormal white blood cell counts. For many individuals with CFS, the white blood cells counts may appear slightly abnormal due to chronic persistent viral or bacterial infections that have triggered the CFS.[2]

Erythrocyte Sedimentation Rate

An erythrocyte sedimentation rate, commonly called "sed rate" or ESR for short, is a simple and inexpensive test. It is basically a measure of the amount of separation between blood cells and the serum, or liquid portion of the blood. A high rate of sedimentation of red blood cells serves as a general indicator of serious pathology. Typically, this test is nonspecific, meaning that it will not provide any more information other than the indication of an abnormal physiological state. It is also seen as a general marker for the level of inflammation in the body and can serve to indicate subtle chronic disease. In the case of CFS, the sed rates are usually low or normal, indicating that blood cells are not separating from the serum.[1] In fact, these abnormally low levels may be the "single most useful test in diagnosis and management" of CFS, according to Dr. David Bell in his book *The Doctor's Guide to Chronic Fatigue Syndrome*.[3] Generally, an abnormally high sedimentation rate would indicate that some other condition besides CFS is occurring.

Chemistry Panels or Screens

Chemistry screens are batteries of different tests combined into one panel to evaluate the functioning of the liver and kidneys and to check for pathologies of the skeletal system and other systems. Chem screens can also test blood glucose levels, as well as status and ratios of electrolytes such as sodium, potassium, calcium, and phosphorous. This panel is a simple tool for ruling out multiple conditions such as diabetes, liver disease, bone pathology, kidney disorders, gout, and metabolic conditions affecting the major elements in the body. Many of these listed conditions can present with fatigue and muscle weakness characteristic of CFS. In CFS, most of these tests come back within normal range, except for liver function tests in some individuals, which seem mildly elevated.[4] Naturopathic physicians view this slight elevation in liver enzymes as an indicator for "liver congestion" and may respond with the use of nutrition, diet therapy, and herbal medicines to boost the liver's ability to continue detoxification. Elevated liver enzymes can also be perceived as indicators that the individual may be exposed to chemicals or toxic substances in the environment for which the liver is compensating. In that case, the aim of therapy would be to identify the toxic agents and remove them from the patient's lifestyle.

Thyroid Panel

Thyroid diseases, and even minor functional thyroid disorders, are relatively common and usually manifest with fatigue as the primary symptom. A thyroid panel should consist of measuring levels of thyroid stimulating hormone (TSH), which indicates pituitary function, free T3, which is active thyroid hormone unbound by proteins, free T4, which is inactive thyroid hormone soon to be converted into T3, and thyroid autoantibodies. In the case of autoimmune thyroiditis, the antibodies will turn up abnormally high. Most other thyroid disease can be detected with the other three tests, without the need for testing autoantibodies. Performing a thyroid panel not only rules out thyroid disorders as a source of fatigue but also provides one aspect of the overall endocrine system function. In CFS, the thyroid panel is usually normal, but some clinicians have observed new developments of thyroid disorders with ongoing or progressive CFS.[3]

Urinalysis

Urinalysis is also a very routine test, usually consisting of a quick submerging of special indicator strips into a sample of urine from the patient. The urinalysis, or UA, is mostly used to eliminate the possibility of genitourinary conditions causing fatigue, mild fever, and general malaise. Subtle urinary tract infections may not present with the typical burning and pain with urination, so they need to be ruled out in most individuals presenting with these symptoms. This test also excludes kidney diseases and collagen vascular disorders.

SPECIALIZED TESTS

For most individuals with CFS, the CBC, Chem screen, Thyroid panel, UA, and ESR tests are sufficient enough to cover the bases. These tests alone can exclude most conditions with similar symptoms, and even some conditions that tend to correlate with CFS. These tests are relatively affordable, compared to more highly specialized tests described later, as they are easily performed with a single blood draw. Another advantage is that the tests are usually covered by most insurance policies since they are considered standard to primary care practice. However, some individuals with more severe CFS, or more complicated health histories and many other symptoms, might choose to receive further laboratory evaluation of their complex illness. In that case, a few other categories of illnesses should be ruled out, and some other aspects of their CFS should be explored in greater detail. The following tests are not as commonly performed. Some can be performed through primary care medical visits, but other may be considered specialized tests, necessitating consultation with a physician in a specific field of medicine. These tests are often more expensive, generally more invasive, and may or may not be covered by third-party payers (insurance plans).

Rheumatoid Factor

Since joint and muscle pain are common to CFS, it becomes important to rule out rheumatic disease, such as rheumatoid arthritis. Unless the individual also has some kind of joint disease, the rheumatoid factor is negative in those with CFS.

Antinuclear Antibody (ANA)

Many autoimmune conditions, such as systemic lupus erythematosis (SLE), can be tested using the antinuclear antibody test. The ANA measures antibodies against the nuclear composition in cells, indicating generalized autoimmunity. Some of these autoimmune conditions, like SLE, Sjögren's, and vasculitis, can present with malaise, weakness, and body pains similar to CFS. According to one CFS researcher, AL Komaroff, a small percentage of those with CFS actually have very low levels of ANA.[4]

Lyme Disease Antibodies

Lyme disease is a cluster of symptoms caused by the Borrelia spirochete transmitted through deer ticks. It can present with joint pain, malaise, severe fatigue, and even some neurological problems. Lyme is generally tested using a serology, an initial ELISA test with a reflex Western Blot to confirm borderline or positive tests. These tests may be important exclusions for individuals living in endemic areas where deer ticks and Lyme disease are common. One limitation of both the ANA and Lyme ELISA tests is that they may show up borderline positive in individuals with CFS,[5] creating unnecessary confusion and anxiety, leading to the need to conduct more tests.

Viral Antibody Titer Testing

As elaborated in the chapter on etiologies for CFS, many viruses have been associated with the development of this condition which often precipitates with a viral illness.[6] However, as these viruses are quite commonly present in the general population, it is difficult to find direct correlations between any one of these viruses and CFS. Instead, CFS is more likely triggered by viral infection in those who already have genetic or environmental predispositions.[7] Evidence for testing the Epstein-Barr virus, human herpes viruses (HHV-6 and HHV-7), retroviruses, and enteroviruses is conflicting or inconclusive. This is partly due to the fact that many healthy individuals can have high titers of some of these viruses without developing the condition of CFS, as in the case of EBV.[8] There is no real evidence that latent viruses can become reactivated to produce the symptoms characteristic of CFS, contrary to what is suggested about HHV.[9] And the evidence for enteroviruses and retroviruses is still preliminary and inconclusive as subsequent studies have yet to confirm the original results.[10,11,12,13,14]

As the evidence for association between viruses and CFS is still conflicting, viral load testing and antibody titers in patients would be expensive and mostly irrelevant. These tests of viral antibody titers are only recommended if the person is undergoing current active viral infection which may be causing her immune dysfunction and chronic fatigue symptoms.

OTHER CONDITIONS CAUSING CHRONIC FATIGUE

Since CFS has overlapping symptoms with several other conditions, it is important not to exclude CFS by selecting the others for diagnosis. The following are guidelines for those conditions that do not exclude a patient from the diagnosis of CFS[1]:

- A condition defined primarily by symptoms, which cannot be confirmed by diagnostic laboratory tests.
- A condition which is currently being treated, but treatment does not resolve the CFS symptoms.
- A condition that occurred and was resolved prior to the onset of CFS.
- Inconclusive physical examination findings or laboratory or imaging tests for other conditions.

In addition, several very common conditions can lead to chronic fatigue, which is different from CFS.[14] These include the following:

- Preexising physical conditions such as diabetes, heart disease, lung disease, inflammation and chronic pain, liver disorders, cancers, multiple sclerosis, and rheumatoid arthritis.
- Prescription drug use including birth control pills, sedatives and tranquilizers, corticosteroids, antihistamines, antiinflammatory drugs, and medications used to lower elevated blood pressure.
- Other health issues such as depression, adrenal fatigue, stress disorders, environmental illness, impaired liver function, immune dysfunction, and food allergies or intolerances.

While there is no one specific diagnostic test used for confirming CFS, many standard routine laboratory tests can at least exclude the possibilities of other conditions causing symptoms of chronic fatigue. In CFS, these tests usually present with normal findings. The difficulty and frustration for many individuals with CFS is that when these tests show normal results, these patients are dismissed as "hypochondriacs" and told that "there is nothing wrong with you." This "all in your head" mentality can be quite disheartening for individuals who just want to understand the cause of their symptomatology. Rather than serve as a measure of disappointment, the lack of positive findings in these tests can actually be the very confirmation of CFS that people are looking for. At that point, it is important to define the condition based on the CDC diagnostic criteria, and ensure that no other ailments or prescriptive drug use are inducing the fatigue. Thorough laboratory evaluation and comprehensive health history by the physician may be the steps needed to make the final solid diagnosis.

CHAPTER 5

Alternative Testing Strategies

The first step in diagnosis of chronic fatigue syndrome (CFS) is for the health-care provider to take a detailed medical history and evaluate whether the person's symptoms match the criteria for CFS. It helps to recognize any connections among all of the factors creating the pattern of illness. It also helps to review past health history, searching for viral infections, periods of intense stress, family history and social environment, medication use, and any other causes for chronic fatigue.

Along with a general physical examination, the important next step is to exclude other health conditions that can mimic the symptoms of chronic fatigue syndrome. If no other health conditions can explain the symptoms, and no other overlapping disorders can be identified, then the diagnosis of CFS is made through exclusion. General laboratory tests that can exclude the most common CFS-like illnesses are the complete blood count, chemistry screen, thyroid panel, urinalysis, and sedimentation rate. For the most part, these tests reveal normal findings in those with chronic fatigue syndrome. So the final diagnosis is made based on meeting the CDC definition criteria for this condition.

While there are no real diagnostic testing strategies in conventional medicine, other than the ones used to exclude the possibility of other diseases, there are some functional tests used in alternative medicine for evaluating certain aspects of CFS. Functional tests are termed such because they can evaluate the overall physiological functioning of the person. These tests do not simply identify whether or not a person has a particular illness. Rather, they can go beyond that. Some of the alternative tests reviewed in this chapter can be used to determine overall state of wellness and specific range of functioning per organ system in the body. When repeated later, they can reveal progress of the condition with treatment. It is important to remember that alternative tests are not meant to officially diagnose chronic fatigue syndrome. Instead these tests are used to understand the complex components of this illness, and the unique manifestation of CFS from one individual to the next.

Several tests used by holistic practitioners are described here for the understanding of the person with CFS. Naturopathic physicians can order and interpret the findings of these types of tests for identifying potential sources of problems and for evaluating efficacy of treatments prescribed to each patient. Unfortunately, many of these tests are not yet integrated into the standard protocol in the Western medical model. As such, they are typically not covered by third-party insurance payers and end up being out-of-pocket expenses. None of these tests are absolutely mandatory to diagnose or treat CFS. So it is not always necessary to use these tests to commence an appropriate and beneficial treatment plan. However, these tests can offer plenty of insight into the workings and dysfunctions of the individual patient, allowing for a more patient-centered individualized therapeutic approach. When used in conjunction with a comprehensive natural approach to therapeutics and follow-up evaluation of these therapeutics for CFS, these tests may prove to be invaluable. The laboratories listed here serve as resources for individuals and practitioners wishing to conduct further evaluation; the author has no vested interest in promoting these laboratories over others.

ADRENAL FUNCTION TESTS

Adrenal, pituitary, and hypothalamic dysfunction are common findings in chronic fatigue syndrome. Overall cortisol production is lowered, possible due to suboptimal function of the hypothalamus or the adrenal glands.[1] This suppressed cortisol output seems to be the worst in the morning, when normal cortisol levels are supposed to be at their peak.[2] Some studies show that it may not be the adrenal glands' fault alone. Inadequate cortisol output might be due to a "blunted" or insufficient output of pituitary hormone adrenocorticotropic hormone (ACTH) in response to hypothalamic prodding of the pituitary gland.[1,3,4,5]

Patterns of neuroendocrine imbalance such as these can be observed through adrenal stress tests, which track the level of hormonal dysfunction in those with chronic fatigue syndrome. One type of measurement is the 24-hour salivary cortisol pattern test. This test measures cortisol and DHEA (another adrenal hormone) from the patient's saliva at selected intervals throughout the day, such as 8 A.M., noon, 5 P.M., and midnight. According to several research studies, salivary measurements may be better indicators of adrenal function than serum (blood) levels.[6,7,8] One major advantage of checking salivary cortisol over cortisol in the serum is that the former does not have to take into account the issue of a protein in the blood called cortisol-binding globulin.[9] So the salivary test measures for free (unbound or available) cortisol.

The adrenal stress test kits offer instructions on how to reduce confounding factors such as dietary interference, oral contaminants, and dental or oral disease.

Regardless of these potential factors, the salivary cortisol and DHEA measurements are excellent markers for gauging the diurnal variations of these hormones. Contrary to so many other conditions in which cortisol levels are too high, CFS is characterized by abnormally low levels throughout the day, especially in the morning, which can be observed with a salivary hormone profile. Results from a 24-hour cortisol test may show evidence of adrenal dysfunction and offer insights into how to direct treatment plans. In an individual with chronically low cortisol output manifesting as fatigue, natural therapeutics can be prescribed to help bolster the body's production of this hormone. On the other hand, an individual whose cortisol levels spike and fall intermittently throughout the 24-hour cycle might be better served with a treatment plan aimed at helping the body modulate the extremes.

While the 24-hour salivary tests are aimed at evaluating levels of cortisol and DHEA, another type of test can be used to ascertain the levels of ACTH. This hormone, released from the pituitary gland to provoke adrenal synthesis of cortisol, is often abnormal in CFS. Like cortisol, ACTH secretion is usually low throughout the day, and especially so in the morning.[5] Pituitary hormones such as this are part of a complex interplay of other biochemical messengers in the body. The use of 24-hour urinary hormone profiles can offer a way of evaluating hypothalamic and pituitary hormones, as well as their metabolites or breakdown products.[6,10] This is one method of determining if the cortisol abnormalities are actually secondary to suboptimal pituitary function. Again, information such as this can influence the therapeutic aim.

Adrenal hormone profiling can be done through one of several laboratories specializing in alternative testing strategies. A health-care practitioner who is trained in the field of alternative or holistic medicine can order and interpret these tests. The laboratories that specialize in adrenal hormone testing are Diagnos-Techs, Inc. (for their salivary Adrenal Stress Index), and ZRT Laboratory (for salivary hormone evaluation tests).

Diagnos-Techs, Inc.
6620 South 192nd Place, Building J
Kent, Washington 98032
(800) 878-3787
www.diagnostechs.com

ZRT Laboratory
8605 SW Creekside Pl.
Beaverton, OR 97008
866-600-1636
www.zrtlab.com

FOOD ALLERGY AND INTESTINAL PERMEABILITY TESTING

The prevalence of allergies and atopy in CFS is becoming more and more obvious. A review article in 1988 found that up to half of the people with CFS also suffered from some degree of atopy.[11] One particular marker for allergies, the eosinophilic cationic protein, is elevated with CFS and may prove to be part of the "common immunologic background" between CFS and atopy.[12] Furthermore, the hyperactive immune function which seems to trigger allergies may also interface with neuroendocrine function.[13]

This allergic picture extends to the issue of food allergies and intolerances as well. A study of 200 individuals with chronic fatigue revealed that many reported multiple intolerances to foods.[14] Intake of food intolerances can stimulate release of various types of cytokines which induce CFS-like symptoms such as fatigue, malaise, headaches, joint pain, and digestive problems.[15] Other clinical studies showed that when individuals with CFS eliminated common food intolerances from their diet, they noticed significant improvement in fatigue, physical depletion, and mental outlook.[16,17] It seems clear that testing for, and implementing a therapeutic diet around, food allergies or intolerances would be a beneficial treatment option for CFS.

The concept of food allergies and food sensitivities which has been around for a few decades is reemerging with the recent surge of medical research around it. Food allergies seem to arise from a problem called intestinal permeability. Normally, the cells lining the intestinal tract provide an effective barrier against excessive absorption of food particles. These food particles are viewed by the immune system as foreign antigens, or substances that initiate an immune reaction against them. When the intestinal cells become excessively permeable, they allow food antigens to cross the barrier, inducing an excessive immune reaction.[18] This immune hyper-response is called a food allergy. Testing for intestinal permeability can provide additional information to the food intolerance issue.

Comprehensive Digestive Stool Analysis

One of the best ways to test for food allergies is to evaluate intestinal permeability.[19,20] According to pioneering naturopaths, Drs. Michael Murray and Joe Pizzorno, "intestinal permeability testing evaluates the small intestine's effectiveness as a macromolecule barrier, monitors changes in mucosal permeability, and determines underlying causes of systemic problems linked to GI function." A comprehensive digestive stool analysis offers a thorough assessment of food allergies caused by intestinal permeability. By carefully examining the digestion and absorption status of the GI tract through a patient's stool sample, evidence can be found for digestive dysfunction: factors showing reduced digestive enzyme secretions, markers for increased intestinal permeability, factors indicating inflammation, and even measurements of the variety of bacterial gut flora and other microorganisms.[21] Laboratories that conduct such studies are Genova Diagnostics (formerly known as Great Smokies Diagnostics Laboratories), which specializes in comprehensive digestive stool analysis tests, and Metametrix Clinical Laboratory for their gastrointestinal function profile tests as well as their salivary hormone panels.

Genova Diagnostics
63 Zillicoa Street,Asheville, NC 28801
(828)253-0621
www.gdx.net

Metametrix Clinical Laboratory
4855 Peachtree Ind. Blvd, Norcross GA 30092
800-221-4640
www.metametrix.com

Secretory IgA

Another method of testing for food allergies is to check levels of secretory IgA. This immunoglobulin protein is secreted in the intestines as a way of defending against any pathogens and foreign substances in the digestive tract.[22] It supports immune reactions to microorganisms like bacteria, viruses, parasites, fungi, and also chemical toxins and food antigens by creating immune complexes around these particles and by preventing them from being absorbed into the cells of the intestine. Secretory IgA is also released into the saliva and other mucosal fluids for this same reason.

Chronically high stress levels that induce abnormal changes in the adrenal endocrine system can significantly reduce sIgA response.[23] When sIgA production is reduced, the mucosal lining is affected and overall tolerance to foods becomes impaired.[21] At this point, when the digestive tract becomes more susceptible to pathogens, the likelihood of developing food allergies increases. The sIgA immunoglobulin can be checked from a blood and/or stool sample. Fecal or stool sIgA testing can reveal subtle food allergies. This is often included in comprehensive digestive stool analysis tests but can also be ordered as a single test from laboratories such as Genova or Metametrix.

Food Allergy Testing

Food allergies can also be tested by reviewing the immunological parameters associated with consuming certain foods. In this type of testing, various immune cells and factors are measured for their stimulation in response to many different foods, inhalants, herbs, and spices. Adverse reactions to foods induce an immunological response in which antibodies are produced. Antibodies, the immune response to food antigens, can be depicted by two special sets of immunoglobulin proteins called IgG and IgE. IgE-mediated food allergies manifest with acute symptoms that occur within minutes up to several hours on ingesting the particular food. When IgE antibodies are activated, they can bind to specific immune cells (mast cells), which create the characteristic symptoms of stomach cramping, diarrhea, skin rash, itching, and even anaphylaxis. The other type of food allergy is mediated through a different group of antibodies called IgG. The symptoms of an IgG-mediated response may occur several hours

Table 5.1. Review of Alternative Testing Strategies

Test	What it checks for	Laboratories performing the tests
Adrenal Stress Index	24-hour salivary cortisol and DHEA levels for assessing adrenal function	Diagnos-Techs, Inc.
Adrenal Hormone Profile	24-hour salivary cortisol and DHEA levels for assessing adrenal function	ZRT Laboratories Metametrix Laboratories
Food Allergy Panels	IgG and IgE antibody reactions to foods, spices, and herbs	US Biotek Alcat Worldwide Metametrix Laboratories Genova Laboratories
Secretory IgA	sIgA levels (and potential food intolerance status)	Diagnos-Techs, Inc.
GI Health Panel	Digestion, enzyme levels, gut immunity markers, bacteria, fungi, yeast, and parasite infection	Diagnos-Techs, Inc.
Comprehensive Digestive Stool Analysis	Digestion, absorption, pancreatic function, inflammation, bacterial balance, yeast, and parasite infection	Genova Laboratories

up to several days after ingestion of the particular food. This delayed food reaction can continue to cause more subtle symptoms lasting for weeks or even months.

Elevations in either of these immunoglobulin proteins (IgG or IgE) may indicate allergic responses to specific foods. When these specific foods are eliminated from the individual's diet, the body will eventually reduce its reactions such that symptoms like tiredness, muscle and joint pain, irritable bowel-like symptoms, and even cognitive dysfunction may resolve.

Several laboratories specialize in the testing of allergies to foods, inhalants, spices, and herbs. These include Metametrix, Genova, US Biotek Laboratories, Alcat Worldwide, and others.

US Biotek Laboratories
13500 Linden Ave North, Seattle WA 98133
877.318.8728
www.usbiotek.com

Alcat Worldwide
1239 E. Newport Center Dr Suite 101, Deerfield Beach FL 33442
800.872.5228
www.alcat.com

Alternative medical tests can be invaluable in revealing the overall phys-iological functioning of each individual. While not necessarily mandatory for diagnosing someone with CFS, these tests often provide clues into aspects of how a person might have developed this condition, how he should be treated, and whether or not a prescribed treatment plan is appropriate and effective. This is yet another way of understanding each person as a unique individual, with his/her own expression of CFS. Table 5.1 provides a summary of the alternative tests, what they evaluate for in a CFS individual, and the names of several laboratories that perform such tests.

PART III

Natural Treatments for Chronic Fatigue Syndrome

CHAPTER 6

Nature Cures—
Alternative Medicine
Modalities

Traditional nature-based medical systems date back thousands of years, from areas all over the world. The healing arts of medicinal herbalism, diet therapies, foods and nutrition, sunlight and mineral and water therapies, acupuncture, homeopathy, spiritualism, shamanism, and intuitive medicines have sustained humans for generations and continue to be used by the majority of the world's population today as primary sources of health care. Regardless of the style and practice, what all of the various healing traditions share is the belief in the healing power of nature. Each living being can return to a state of resilient equilibrium due to an intrinsic ability to heal. When disease arises from a disruption in the normal function, recovery occurs naturally by the individual either unassisted or through therapy based on natural remedies. Nature cures. And it is the healer's role to guide this healing process.

A renewed appreciation in this philosophy, and in the variety of medical systems that promote this perspective, has recently emerged. In response to the popularity and increasing use of these modalities, the National Institutes of Health (NIH) created the National Center for Complementary and Alternative Medicine in 1998 to fund research into alternative medicine for a better understanding of its efficacy. Complementary and alternative medicine (CAM) was a term coined around that time to encompass the many different modalities of natural medicines originating from around the world commonly used in practice today in the United States. It seems ironic to call these natural medicine modalities "complementary" or "alternative" as they have such a rich and universal history of use and as they continue to be used in primary health care globally today. Nevertheless, these nature-based healing practices are of great interest for their noninvasiveness, effectiveness in treatment with minimal side effects, and promotion of self-empowerment for health.

Alternative medicine therapies are important options to consider when dealing with conditions whose etiologies are multifactorial. Most chronic illness with multiple cause and triggers require fresh perspectives and interdisciplinary therapeutic approaches to allow more than one medical system to overlap and to offer the benefits of variety and synergy in treatments. In the case of chronic fatigue syndrome (CFS), no single drug treatment is available, and conventional medicine has limitations to its effectiveness. Only cognitive behavior therapy and graded exercise therapies have shown solid evidence for efficacy thus far.[1] A systematic review of the scientific literature by Whiting et al. suggests that pharmaceutical medication therapy, such as immunoglobulin and hydrocortisone, have "limited effects" and that the clinical and research-based "evidence is inconclusive." Western medicine has not revealed real solutions yet.

Based on the holistic perspective, alternative medicine practices and therapies can provide individualized, practical, and comprehensive treatment strategies.[2,3] The research on alternative medical approaches to CFS is still relatively new but supportive to the use of natural therapeutics for treatment of this condition. Whiting et al. suggest that this research is still "insufficient" and recommend further research to support even the therapies proven to be effective. In actuality, the current research reveals promising results. What is even more promising is the rich historical foundation from which alternative therapeutics have evolved. Some of these alternative medicine modalities are reviewed here for their approach and for their beneficial use in treatment of CFS.

NATUROPATHIC MEDICINE

Naturopathic medicine is a unique eclectic form of primary care medicine, which incorporates a holistic perspective and integrates a variety of nature-based therapies for the treatment and prevention of disease. The roots of naturopathic medicine can be traced back to a variety of healing traditions from around the world.[4] Its very name comes from the word roots for "nature" and "disease" implying the use of natural modalities for treatment of illness. Naturopathic medicine is based on the premises of optimizing healthy functioning to prevent future disease and empowering each patient to own responsibility for her health.[5]

A true example of holistic medicine, naturopathy is defined not by its treatment modalities, but by six guiding principles. These principles guide each naturopathic physician to follow a common philosophy of treatment, one that focuses on the patient's unique needs and healing abilities.[6]

- *Vis Medicatrix Naturae*—The "healing power of nature" is the inherent healing ability of living beings that maintains and restores health. The role of the naturopathic physician is to remove obstacles to recovery by supporting the individual's vitality and providing a healthy environment for recovery to occur.
- *Tolle Causam*—Identify and treat the causes. The underlying cause of disease must be identified and removed for healing to occur. Symptoms

are expressions of the body's attempt to adapt and recover, or they may be manifestations of the disease process itself. The naturopathic physician seeks to address the root causes of disease, rather than to merely suppress or mask the symptoms.

- *Primum Non Nocere*—First do no harm. Naturopathic physicians utilize methods and medicinal substances that minimize the risk of harmful effects, and apply the least possible force or intervention necessary to diagnose illness and restore health.
- *Docere*—The word "doctor" means one who teaches. A principal objective of the naturopathic doctor is to educate the patient and emphasize self-responsibility for health. The therapeutic relationship between the doctor and the patient is vital for fostering guidance and education needed for patients to feel empowered about making healthful life choices.
- *Treat the whole person as a unique individual*—Health and disease result from a complex of physical, mental, emotional, spiritual, genetic, environmental, and social factors. The complex harmonious interplay of these factors determines the uniqueness of each individual. As such, each individual requires a comprehensive and personalized approach to diagnosis and treatment. Understanding the interface of these factors helps naturopathic doctors treat the whole person, rather than a sum of the parts.
- *Prevention*—Optimizing wellness can help prevent disease in the future. In addition to promoting overall health, naturopathic physicians assess risk factors, heredity, and susceptibility to disease to setup interventions for preventing illness.

Naturopathic physicians (NDs) are considered general practitioners of alternative medicine. They are licensed in many states (and nations around the world) as primary care and specialty doctors who address the underlying cause of disease through effective, individualized natural therapies that integrate the healing powers of body, mind, and spirit. They "integrate scientific research with the healing powers of nature", using therapies that support and promote the body's natural healing process, leading to the highest state of wellness. Many NDs participate in and contribute to the growing body of scientific research to further advance the understanding of natural medicines. Their training in conventional medicine theory allows for a comprehensive understanding in "clinical sciences and the biological basis of healing."[7] This foundation, along with the holistic guiding principles, provides opportunity for an expanded perspective on treating patients. As NDs work with conventionally trained physicians, specialists, and other alternative medical practitioners to co-manage patient care, they continue to evolve the current medical paradigm. According to some physicians, "Naturopathic medicine is an emerging field in one of medicine's most dynamic eras, one that is richer for the inclusion of CAM."[8] In fact, nearly 40 percent of family medicine departments offer some CAM curriculum,[9] including the education about a variety of healing modalities used by naturopathic physicians for centuries.

Naturopathic doctors are the only primary care physicians clinically trained in the use of the following wide variety of natural therapeutics:

Clinical Nutrition: Naturopathic physicians understand that dietary factors are fundamental to health. Adopting a healthy diet is often the first step toward correcting health problems. Many medical conditions can be treated more effectively with foods and nutritional supplements than they can by other means, but with fewer complications and side effects. Naturopathic physicians may use specific individual diets, fasting, and nutritional supplements with their patients.

Botanical Medicine: Plants have powerful healing properties. Many pharmaceutical drugs have their origins in plant substances. Naturopathic physicians use plant substances for their healing effects and nutritional value.

Homeopathic Medicine: This gentle yet effective system of medicine is more than 200 years old and is based on the principle that "Like cures Like." Homeopathic medicines are very small doses of natural substances that can stimulate the body's self-healing response without side effects. These medicines are prepared by a specific process of diluting and potentiating substances to achieve therapeutic value. Some conditions for which conventional medicine has no effective treatments respond well to homeopathy.

Physical Medicine: Naturopathic medicine includes various methods of therapeutic manipulation for muscles and bones. Naturopathic physicians also employ therapeutic exercise, massage, hydrotherapy, gentle electrical therapies, ultrasound, and heat and cold for treatment of pain disorders and inflammation. Hydrotherapy encompasses various traditions and techniques for using water, often in the forms of steam or ice, in noninvasive economically viable ways to stimulate the vital force.

Lifestyle Counseling and Stress Management: Mental attitudes and emotional states can be important elements in healing and disease. Naturopathic physicians are trained in counseling, nutritional balancing, stress management, hypnotherapy, and biofeedback. They also attend to environmental and lifestyle factors that affect their patients' health.

Several of these therapeutic modalities are described in great detail in later chapters for their use in the treatment of CFS. These include, but are not limited to, the use of proper diet and eating habits, supplementation with nutrients, therapeutic use of herbal medicines, and guidelines for exercise and stress reduction for everyday life. These types of therapeutics have proven themselves through research and through historical use in traditional medicines to be highly effective in the treatment of CFS. These therapies can provide support for improving immune function, stress resilience and resistance to oxidative damage, and many other benefits such as improved nutritional status, hormone balancing, and cognitive enhancement. The synergy of using the correct tools (natural medicines) with the appropriate methods (holistic philosophy) offers optimal treatment outcomes with the least potential for harm. While many forms of natural medicines can be safely administered at home for self-treatment, it is advised and strongly encouraged to seek the guidance of a trained physician or health-care professional with expertise in the fields of natural medicines. A list of rigorously trained, licensed naturopathic physicians can be found through the American Association of Naturopathic Physicians online at www.naturopathic.org. Listings for holistic health care practitioners and organizations are provided in the Resources pages.

INTRAVENOUS NUTRIENT THERAPY

The best and most convenient approach to nutrition is through proper intake of nourishing foods in a well-balanced diet rich with a variety of different foods. Because of the abundance of foods available in the United States, severe nutrient deficiencies are rare. However, subclinical or marginal deficiencies are relatively common.[10] Marginal deficiencies may arise from years of imbalanced diets full of processed foods and empty calories. Deficiencies can also arise out of disease states, chronic infections, or long-term use of a variety of medications including prescriptive hormones. Diagnosis of marginal nutrient deficiencies is difficult and costly, involving very detailed analyses of the diet as well as multiple laboratory tests. While most marginal nutritional deficiencies do not create active illness or disease, they do lead up to issues of chronic disease, characterized by symptoms of fatigue, vague musculoskeletal and joint pains, low moods, lack of focus, difficult concentration, and others. In other words, symptoms of nutritional deficiencies dramatically overlap those of CFS and other chronic disorders!

In order to prevent and treat minor deficiencies, it is useful to supplement the diet with good quality multivitamin and mineral formulas tested for purity and quality, which are not full of preservatives and additives and other unwanted particulates. An entire chapter on nutrients has been dedicated to this therapeutic approach. For many who already deal with CFS or other long-term illness, the recommended dosages of some of the nutrients for treatment go way beyond the Recommended Daily Allowance levels (RDA values). Therapeutic levels of nutrients may need to be several times more concentrated than the values suggested for preventing frank disease. While these optimal amounts may be attainable by some, they may be too high to absorb for others.

Intravenous nutrient therapy (IV therapy) is an ideal option for achieving optimal or therapeutic dosages of nutrients, especially in individuals suffering from chronic illness. Nutrients administered intravenously are injected directly into a vein in the forearm or hand by a health-care professional who is trained in the administration of IV therapy. The intravenous injections quickly deliver high concentrations of nutrients directly into the bloodstream for direct action.[11] IV administration of nutrients bypasses the body's entire digestive system, reducing the potential pitfalls that the nutrients will not get broken down or absorbed properly through this system. This method also avoids the possibility of the liver and kidneys metabolizing or excreting the nutrients before the body has a chance to use them. Instead, at high concentrations in the bloodstream, the nutrients circulate throughout the body, depositing into tissues and eventually into cells where they are used for biochemical reactions that sustain functions. When nutrients are present in relatively high concentrations outside the cells (or in the blood stream) compared to inside the cells, they are more readily taken up by the cells. In this way, "IV nutrient therapy may be more effective than oral or intramuscular treatment for correcting intracellular nutrient deficiencies" according to holistic physician Dr. Alan Gaby.[11]

According to this author, and as observed in many different clinical experiences, the use of IV therapy to deliver nutrients has several benefits over oral supplementation and even intramuscular injections. For one, the nutrient levels required to achieve a "pharmaceutical" action during treatment of disease can sometimes be staggering. Even when supplementing the diet, the concentration of the nutrient reaches an upper limit in the blood. This is because the absorption in the gastrointestinal tract achieves its peak saturation, and any amounts over that limit will then be cleared away through the organs of elimination. For example, a twelvefold increase in vitamin C with oral dosing (from 200 mg to 2,500 mg daily) only raises this nutrient's concentration in the blood by 25 percent.[12] The rest is probably flushed out of the body, or just not absorbed at all. Similarly, oral supplementation of magnesium barely increases blood levels of this nutrient. Instead, IV administration can double or even triple the concentrations of these nutrients in the blood for peak therapeutic action.[13] The levels required for certain therapeutic actions might only be achieved through intravenous delivery.

A second reason for IV therapy's superiority over oral and intramuscular administration is that it can be given when there are problems with absorption of nutrition. In genetic disorders affecting the ability to maintain adequate concentrations of nutrients within cells, in conditions where the digestive system is incapable of absorbing nutrients, and in diseases causing the kidneys to rapidly clear out important nutrients, IV therapy may be beneficial and even necessary. Nutrient levels may stay high only transiently in the blood stream, but even in that short period, their levels are high enough to flood into cells. When repeatedly delivered over time, the cells are constantly deluged with the high levels of nutrients, and the overall "improvement may be cumulative" according to Dr. Gaby.

Many different nutrients, and even some botanical extracts, may be given intravenously to treat chronic conditions. While some of these nutrients are given singly, most are combined into specific formulations for the synergistic effect and totality of the treatment. One such combination formula has received some attention for its ability to achieve marked clinical improvement in a variety of conditions. The "Myers' cocktail" was named after the late Dr. John Myers who incorporated intravenous administration of nutrients into his practice. The Myers' cocktail consists of magnesium, calcium, vitamin B complex, and vitamin

C- nutrients shown to be quite beneficial in the treatment of CFS. It is used to treat a variety of other conditions as well, such as asthma, migraine headaches, fibromyalgia, muscle spasms, cardiovascular disease, respiratory tract infections, and many others. In one outpatient study, this therapy was given to about 1,000 individuals who overall showed "marked clinical improvement."[11] Even healthy individuals elected to receive this treatment periodically to support their sense of well-being for months at a time.

The Myer's cocktail of nutrients has been studied in several individuals with CFS.[11] In ten individuals with CFS receiving at least four treatments, distributed once weekly for 1 month, more than half showed improvement. Usually it took three or four injections for them to notice clinical improvement, but one individual enjoyed "dramatic benefit" after the first intravenous injection. Many were able to stop the treatments after a while due to feeling "progressively healthier." Others who did not completely overcome their fatigue still achieved better functioning overall. The research behind the different nutrients used is presented in a following chapter for review. In summary, magnesium, vitamin C, and various B vitamins have all demonstrated significant clinical effectiveness in treatment of people with CFS. In addition to the Myers' cocktail, many other formulations can be designed, with the individual in mind, to contain other beneficial nutrients such as antioxidants, zinc, selenium, CoQ10, L-carnitine, and others.

It takes a good deal of knowledge about the chemical effects of various nutrients, as well as their ability to mix well together, to successfully administer an intravenous formula. Proper administration of IV nutrients also requires skill and practice to perform. Many naturopathic physicians and holistic medical providers are licensed, trained, and certified to provide this therapeutic modality in an outpatient clinical setting. Check the American Association of Naturopathic Physicians, or the state naturopathic physicians association to find an ND trained in the use of intravenous therapy for treatment of CFS.

HOMEOPATHY

The term *homeopathy* is derived from the Greek words *homeos*, meaning "similar," and *pathos*, meaning "suffering." The medicines are chosen based on the philosophy of the Law of Similars (the concept of like curing like). This fundamental homeopathic tenet came forth with the "observed relationship between a medicine's ability to produce a specific constellation of signs and symptoms in a healthy individual and the same medicine's ability to cure a sick patient with similar signs and symptoms."[14] It is thought that Hippocrates himself first recognized that herbs given in low doses tended to cure the same symptoms they produced when given in toxic doses.

Homeopathic medicine is a gentle yet effective system of medicine developed over 200 years ago by a German physician named Samuel Hahnemann. Dr. Hahnemann discovered that when a substance is given in specific dosages, it can produce a predictable pattern of physical, biochemical, and mental-emotional outcomes. He also observed that the same substance prepared in minute doses would actually "cure" the very effects induced by larger dosages. In other words, clinical symptoms arising from large dosages of particular medicines could be reversed and treated using the same substance in diluted form. Because of this effect, virtually any condition with a certain specific set of signs and symptoms can be treated with a specific homeopathic medicine. This principle of "Like cures Like" frames the premise for why homeopathy works and how it is used. Samuel Hahnemann continued to research and explore this technique in his practice to cure many individuals afflicted with infectious disease and chronic disorders. Today, homeopathic medicines are used in countries all over the world, including the United States, to promote healing and wellness, and recovery from disease.

Remedies prepared as homeopathic medicines are very small doses of natural substances that can stimulate the body's self-healing response without side effects. The homeopathic approach does not combat disease symptoms in the same manner as one would in conventional practice. Instead, homeopathic philosophy states that if the person is brought back into balance, the symptoms of disease (imbalance) will resolve accordingly. A homeopathic physician looks for a broad and unique picture of imbalance specific to each person. Some conditions for which conventional medicine has no effective treatments may respond well to homeopathy. A meta-analysis published in the *British Medical Journal* of a total of 105 controlled trials showed positive results for homeopathic treatment in eighty-one trials, leading its authors to state, "The evidence in this review would probably be sufficient for establishing homeopathy as a regular treatment for certain indications."[15]

Preliminary evidence supports benefits and effectiveness of homeopathy for treatment of CFS. Several homeopathic case reports of successful outcomes in patients with CFS have been published.[16] In one clinical trial, a multitherapeutic approach was embraced to treat eighty-one individuals with CFS.[17] These individuals were treated with a wheat-free diet, nutritional supplements, and unique homeopathic constitutional treatments over several months, with each different phase of treatment added in monthly intervals. Seventy percent of those completing the study showed positive improvement overall! The researchers observed improvement with each treatment intervention, and each improvement continued even after introduction of a different treatment. Now this study has one important limitation. Because of the multifactorial nature of the various treatment modalities used, it is difficult to figure out the exact individual benefits for each treatment used. However, as a pilot or preliminary study, it shows great opportunity to continue research into the use of homeopathic medicines as one aspect of treatment. It also provided the information that there were no side effects for homeopathy, and instead that the patients definitely showed signs of improvement. It will be interesting to find out what more these researchers reveal in the future.

Another study used a triple-blind approach for evaluating the effects of homeopathic medicine on those with CFS.[18] "Triple-blind" means that the subjects, their homeopathic physicians, and the data analysts were not given any information about one another to avoid bias in the results. Forty-seven individuals with CFS had monthly consults with their homeopathic physicians for a total of 6 months during which time homeopathic medicines unique to each individual's needs were given. Evaluation consisted of several fatigue inventories and limitation profiles. Those who received customized homeopathic formulas experienced significantly greater improvement in the fatigue and physical limitation profiles. In addition, more people receiving homeopathic medications showed minor but definite improvement on all primary outcome measures. The authors concluded that, although not as significant as they would have liked to see, the evidence supported that homeopathic medicine was superior to placebo in treatment of individuals with CFS. Another double-blind trial in the United Kingdom found that one-third of the sixty-four patients with CFS experienced significant improvement compared to almost no one from the placebo group. This is indeed a fascinating approach to treatment for those with CFS, and future clinical trials might continue to find some dramatic positive benefits.[19]

The practice of homeopathic medicine is very much an art. It involves a thorough and comprehensive interview, case analysis, and the ability to prescribe a single homeopathic remedy based on a totality of symptoms for each individual. Contrary to the "one size fits all" approach so common in allopathic medicine, homeopathic physicians select just one remedy at a time to address the most unique attributes of each individual patient. Because of this philosophy, it takes time and presence of mind to thoroughly listen to each patient's needs and challenges. It also means that there is no single homeopathic remedy to treat everyone with CFS. So unfortunately, none are recommended for universal support of fatigue. Instead, it is recommended to seek the care of a well-trained homeopathic practitioner for consultation and prescription of the correct homeopathic medicine for the person dealing with CFS. The North American Society of Homeopaths is a solid resource for learning more about homeopathy and locating a trained, licensed, or certified homeopathic practitioner. In addition, naturopathic physicians are trained in the use of homeopathic medicines and many are considered experts in this field. For a resource on NDs also practicing homeopathy, refer to the American Association of Naturopathic Physicians as well.

AYURVEDIC MEDICINE

Ayurvedic medicine evolved in ancient India almost 6,000 years ago, since around 4,500 B.C. This medical tradition is still revered in many countries and cultures, and still practiced today as a form of primary health care for many. The name is derived from the Sanskrit language meaning "the science of life" from *ayus* (life) and *veda* (knowledge).[20] As such, the focus is on establishing and maintaining balance of the life energies within each individual, rather than focusing on individual symptoms. In Ayurveda, each person has his own constitution type, or a unique set of characteristics that reveal his physiological and genetic makeup. Although two people may appear to have the same outward symptoms, each person has energetic constitutions that may be very different from the other. Therefore each calls for very different treatment plans. This understanding of the unique constitutional differences of all individuals allows an ayurvedic practitioner to design treatment recommendations to fit the particular constitution.

The goal of Ayurveda is to assist natural healing processes by promoting harmony between the individual and his/her environment and by supporting a lifestyle of balance. Ayurveda seeks to restore wholeness and harmony to people through proper nutrition, lifestyle, and herbal medicines. Ayurvedic treatment involves detoxification therapies, botanicals, oil massage treatments, and diet and lifestyle changes. Any or all of the treatments may be chosen, based on the condition of the patient and the severity of ailment. For long-term prevention, diet, nutrition, and herbal medicine routines are custom designed and prescribed as overall lifestyle changes. These treatments have been shown to be safe and effective in treating many chronic ailments.[20,21] Beyond the diet and herbal medicine aspects to health, the primary underlying basis of Ayurveda is actually a spiritual foundation—one that reminds us to settle the mind and regularly work toward a more conscious lifestyle.

From an ayurvedic standpoint, disease arises from an imbalance in the three *doshas*, or biomaterials, which the body is made up of. These primary elements of *vata (air and ether)*, *pitta (fire)*, and *kapha (earth and water)* in proper, balanced levels can ensure good health[22] similar to the modern day medical philosophy of homeostasis, or the state of biochemical and physiological equilibrium. But disturbances in this state of equilibrium over time can lead to disease. CFS is diagnosed in Ayurveda as deficiency of body strength and vitality due to inadequate assimilation of nutrients and metabolism to make energy.[23] According to one ayurvedic physician, Dr. Sivarama Vinjamury, the basic treatment consists of "tonifying herbs and maintenance of proper digestive function."

A case report shows how Ayurvedic principles and treatment helped one woman with CFS overcome her condition.[23] She was treated with a botanical formula consisting of adaptogenic herbs that would support her body's resistance to stress. She was also given a gooseberry jam called "Chyawanprash" containing herbs and minerals for improving her body's energy, hormonal balance, and metabolism of nutrients. Dietary changes included eliminating fried foods, soda, and specific vegetables that seemed to aggravate her digestive system. Other lifestyle changes included breathing exercises to reduce the effects of stress. The patient reported significant symptomatic improvement based on fatigue impact scales, sleep questionnaires, and cognitive functioning profiles. After just 2 months of treatment, she was noticing less fatigue, increased energy, and improved ability to exercise regularly without pain or postexertional burnout. The scientific and medical basis for the herbs and nutrients used are reviewed in detail in the chapter on botanical medicines.

Promising results like these give credit to the use of and further study of ayurvedic treatments for CFS. Larger randomized controlled clinical trials are needed to evaluate efficacy of this type of treatment, using individualized approaches to therapy for each volunteer presenting with CFS. Dr. Vinjamury recommends a "staged approach" to developing a research trial to ensure that the complexity of treatment is not lost in the research process. So far, many plant-based therapies commonly used in Ayurveda have been studied for their efficacy in the treatment of a variety of chronic ailments.[24] Many plant medicines have been studied in humans and other animals, showing support in their use as medicines for various conditions.[25] In addition, there is some evidence to support the physiological differences among the different constitution types by explaining them in terms of the free radical approach to disease.[26] This gives credibility to the theory of different constitution types in Ayurveda from a biochemical perspective, helping integrate this ancient philosophy into modern scientific medicine.

A good resource for finding a qualified ayurvedic physician is through the National Ayurvedic Medical Association. An Ayurvedic physician will likely conduct a thorough medical and psychological history for evaluating the causes of CFS, paying special attention to symptoms of depression, self-destructive thought processes, psychomotor retardation, and evidence of neurological or psychological disorders. From there, physical examination may also include diagnosis based on the appearance and palpation of the tongue and pulse. The prescribed treatments will be designed for the individual, including dietary recommendations, botanical medicinal formulations, lifestyle suggestions, and detoxification therapies based on the discretion of the provider and compliance of the patient.

CHINESE MEDICINE AND ACUPUNCTURE

Chinese medicine dates back to around 5,000 years ago, beginning with a legend about the Yellow Emperor Huangdi (circa 2698 to 2598). As the "father of Chinese medicine," Huangdi wrote one of the oldest texts, the Canon of Medicine.[27] Thus began a tradition of medicine with links to medicinal therapies evolving in India at that time. It is based on a theory that health relies on the proper flow of energy through the body. This energy, also called Qi (pronounced "chi"), courses throughout the living being and defines the very essence of life itself. Disease is caused by the lack of proper Qi flow in the system, resulting in pain due to stagnation and other ailments due to improper functioning.

Chinese medicine theory is also based on the concepts of the five elements (fire, metal, earth, wood, and water) as well as the duality of Yin and Yang. All diagnoses and treatments are based on the five element theory and on the balance of Yin and Yang, which represent male and female energies in their most reductionistic explanation. In perfect balance, in optimal health, Yin and Yang are harmonious, like the ebb and flow of the tides, like day and night, like male and female. Whenever one or the other presents as deficiency or excess, pathology ensues, manifesting with symptoms such as pain, fatigue, indigestion, poor sleep, mood disorders, and many others.[28]

Chinese medicine is a comprehensive system involving the use of diet therapy, herbal medicines, balanced lifestyle, and acupuncture. The official definition of acupuncture by the NIH is "a family of procedures involving stimulations of anatomical locations on the skin by a variety of techniques, [including] penetration of the skin by thin, solid, metallic needles."[29] The insertion of these fine needles is understood to open gates for the correct flow of energy throughout the body. When inserted along specific body points called "meridians," they can stimulate or support the vital function of various organs. By stimulating these points, a person's "vital energy," or "Qi," can be balanced and restored. Acupuncture is used to relieve pain, prevent nausea, and to treat substance abuse as well as many other conditions. Because acupuncture needles are sterile and used only once before being properly discarded, side effects are rare and minimal.

A couple of clinical trials have presented solid results for the efficacy of acupuncture and Chinese herbal medicine in the treatment of CFS. In one recent study, forty-six patients, whose ages ranged from 19 to 44, composed of more men than women, were treated with a Chinese herbal preparation called *bu gan yi qi tang,* composed of multiple botanicals in root, seed, and other forms.[30] After several courses of treatment, almost 25 percent of the volunteers noted some improvement in symptoms such as extreme fatigue, insomnia, depression, and lack of strength. The remaining three-quarters of the group actually experienced complete abatement of their symptoms! In another pilot study of adolescents, acupuncture seemed to show great benefit.[31] Eight pediatric patients with CFS ranging from ages 11 to 18 were treated with acupuncture once weekly for 6 weeks. They had originally complained of loss of concentration (75%), low school attendance (75%), unrefreshing sleep (75%), pain in the back (75%), joint pain (75%), neck pain (75%), headache (75%), dizziness (50%), depression (50%), bowel dysfunction (50%), abdominal pain (50%), orthostatic hypotension (50%), and mood disorder (38%). After just one treatment, many reported falling asleep faster and feeling more energy afterward. And after the full course of treatment, all were able to return to school. Even though their baseline scores for fatigue, sleep, and functioning levels did not change significantly, the clinical improvements were remarkable and the duration of effectiveness lasted longer after each subsequent treatment. Although there is no one theory in Chinese medicine to explain the disease mechanism of CFS for everyone, the core philosophy is that of "liver-spleen disharmony."[32] This is thought to be due to things like poor diet, excessive thinking and anxiety, overwork, inadequate amounts of exercise, and overuse of cold bitter medicinals such as antibiotics. In addition to acupuncture and medicinal herbs, Chinese medicine advocates a healthier lifestyle for people with CFS to counteract the effects of overwork, mental exhaustion, and eating a poor diet. Like many other alternative medicine practices, Chinese medicine and acupuncture show promising results for those with CFS.

Chinese medicine and acupuncture have become very popular alternative medicine modalities, especially in the United States, over the past few decades. Several research studies and clinical trials support its efficacy in a variety of different conditions. According to the NIH, acupuncture is "an acceptable alternative, or part of a comprehensive treatment program."[29] In practice, an acupuncturist will take a detailed family history of health and illness and ask questions about past minor ailments, personal traits, preferences, and habits. He/she will use palpation of the pulse and examination of the tongue as primary diagnostic tools to evaluate the flow of Qi through the meridians and normal functioning of the organ systems. Like most alternative medical practices, the goal is to restore health and well-being by eliminating the roots of the problem. Each treatment is individualized to fit the needs of the patient, and it may take at least four to five treatments for noticeable improvement to occur. A good resource for locating a trained licensed acupuncturist and Chinese medicine practitioner is at the American Association of Oriental Medicine.

ALTERNATIVE MEDICINE FOR CFS

So far, the modern medicine model of treatment for CFS is limited to cognitive behavior therapy and graded exercise therapy. These modalities may be very effective for some, but do not necessarily address the true multifactorial and complex nature of CFS. In fact, the scientific and medical communities have yet to agree on any pharmaceutical prescriptions for CFS sufferers that are reliable and universal and effective. It is time to shift our focus from a "one size fits all" model to one of individualized patient-centered wellness and health empowerment. Medical practices from around the world that have been termed "complementary" or "alternative" are more commonly taking the lead role in the treatment of long-term debilitating disease. For those suffering from chronic illness for which the conventional treatment options are limited or inadequate, alternative medicine has become more of a primary source of health care. Naturopathic medicine, homeopathy, ayurvedic medicine, Chinese medicine, and numerous other healing traditions all share a common holistic philosophy of treating the individual as a whole, using remedies found in nature, and supporting the individual's own healing process through diet and lifestyle factors. When it comes to treating someone with CFS, a holistic medical philosophy that embraces the patterns found in nature can best address the overlap between nuances of each unique individual and the real complexities of this condition.

CHAPTER 7

Mind, Body, and Lifestyle

The best therapeutic plans for most illnesses can be established right at home. When diseases arise from improper functioning of the body, we must begin from within to correct the imbalance. Each individual holds his/her own cure to his/her health problems. This personal journey to cure starts with a healthful diet filled with nourishing foods, regular physical activity, time for emotional reflection and personal growth, and support from community. Individuals suffering from CFS must consider creating a lifestyle that nourishes the mind and body together, in simple everyday ways.

FOOD, DIET, AND NOURISHMENT

The old adage "You are what you eat" rings true about the effect of diet on health. Hippocrates, considered one of the founders of modern medicine, advised from the very beginning that food is our best medicine. To achieve good health, it is vital to nourish the body with healthful foods. This is true for those who are healthy as well as those who are suffering from illness or disease. The body can only enjoy the benefits of exuberant energy when it is appropriately fueled. For those suffering from chronic fatigue syndrome (CFS), it is even more important to take in a nourishing diet. This can reduce the progress of this condition as well as support the body's own healing process for achieving optimal wellness.

In CFS, when energy levels and overall functioning of the body are down, the diet needs to provide lots of nutrition in the forms of macronutrients (carbohydrates, proteins, and fats) as well as micronutrients (vitamins, minerals, enzymes, and others). While charging the physical body with vital foods, it is also important to avoid consuming foods and other products that drain the body of its energy and resources. A whole foods diet, full of fresh fruits and vegetables and legumes, whole grains, nuts and seeds and small amounts of lean meats, healthful fats, and minimal processed foods is the best recommendation. In fact, the following dietary guidelines for supporting health in CFS are universal for anyone wishing to optimize their wellness. Some of these general healthy diet guidelines are inspired from a wonderful reference text for natural medicine written by two eminent naturopathic physicians: The Textbook of Natural Medicine by doctors Michael Murray, ND, and Joseph Pizzorno, ND.[1]

MACRONUTRIENTS: CARBOHYDRATES, PROTEINS, FATS, WATER

Carbohydrates

Recently, with the emergence of many fad diets in our culture, the idea of eating carbohydrates has become virtually unthinkable. "Carbs" have become synonymous with weight gain and are considered a major taboo according to some popular weight loss diets. This is unfortunate since carbohydrates actually offer so many benefits in the diet, including providing a major source of energy for all body functions.

Carbohydrates can be divided into one of two categories: complex and simple carbohydrates. Complex carbohydrates are made of long chains of sugars called monosaccharides. Bound up with these long chains of sugars are fibers that make up some of the bulk in fruits, vegetables, legumes, and whole grains. These fibers are either in the form of celluloses and pectins in vegetables, legumes, and fruits, or the germ and the bran in whole grains before they are milled. The bran is the layer that covers the grain kernels and contains fiber as well as proteins and trace minerals. The germ is the growing part of the grain, which provides most of the B Vitamins, trace minerals, essential fatty acids, and Vitamin E.[2] Sadly, the milling and refining process removes many of these important nutrients and fibers from the grain, leaving whole grains superior food products compared to refined grains. Whole grains include whole wheat, brown rice, teff, quinoa, cous-cous, oats, barley, millet, rye, and many others. The cellulose fibers found in vegetables provide structure and support for the plant. These types of fibers cannot be broken down by the human digestive process, and are termed "insoluble fibers." They stimulate digestive tract motility, increase the bulk of stools, and can even dilute the concentration of toxic compounds that need to be excreted from the bowels.[2] The pectins and gums found in plant-based foods comprise the group called "soluble fibers," which help to bind bile salts for excretion and support the growth and balance of beneficial bacteria in the colon. Together, the insoluble and soluble fibers in fruits, vegetables, and whole grains offer the overall health benefits of complex carbohydrates. Among these health benefits are: improved insulin sensitivity to control and prevent diabetes,[3] increased binding and excretion of bile salts which lowers cholesterol,[4] and the prevention and treatment of a variety of medical conditions such as cancers, obesity, cardiovascular disease, diabetes, and gastrointestinal disorders.[5]

Simple carbohydrates include simple sugars that are found in fruits, milk products, most sweeteners, and in most processed food. While some of these substances are found in nature, such as honey, fruit sugars, lactose in milk, and others, many are derived by refining and milling out the germ and fibers normally bound to the original carbohydrate. The problem with simple carbohydrates is that they are rapidly absorbed into the bloodstream, creating a very quick rise in blood sugar levels. In response, the body releases insulin to control for the high blood sugar levels, and over time this dramatic peak and fall causes a strain on the body's metabolism, leading to conditions associated with insulin resistance such as diabetes. When complex carbohydrates are refined to produce simple carbohydrates, such as white flour, white sugars, and even breakfast cereals, much of the original vitamins and minerals are removed. This leaves a commercial product that provides the sugar rush but lacks the nutritional value, appropriately named an "empty calorie food." Unfortunately, over half the carbohydrates consumed in the United States fall under this category of simple sugars in processed foods.[5]

For individuals suffering from CFS, it is especially important to take in nutritional components in complex carbohydrate foods, while avoiding the rapid sugar rise from eating processed foods high in simple sugars. Eating a diet rich in whole grains, vegetables, and fruits can provide the much-needed vitamins, minerals, and fiber necessary for energy and proper physiological functioning across multiple organ systems. It is highly recommended to avoid refined simple carbohydrates and to beware of products containing empty calories found in sucrose, glucose, maltose, lactose, fructose, corn syrup, or white grape juice concentrate. For most adults, the complex carbohydrate portion of the diet should amount to 50 to 70 percent of the total daily calories. A nutritionist or healthcare provider specializing in nutrition can provide more individualized guidance as needed.

Proteins

Proteins are considered to be the building blocks of life. These macronutrients are invaluable in the body for producing tissues, muscles, bone, enzymes, and even immune cells, like antibodies, and certain hormones, like insulin. They are required in large amounts during times of stress and injury for their ability to repair cells and tissues, and they maintain normal structural components. In addition, proteins can be broken down during periods of starvation to release simple sugar components needed for energy sources. So in terms of optimizing health and preventing disease, proteins serve to provide much nutritional value. In fact, one of the most prominent advantages of proteins in the diet is their ability to stabilize the effect on blood sugar levels.[2] Adequate amounts of good quality protein in the diet curbs the effects of rapid rise and fall of blood sugar from carbohydrates in the diet.

Because the body can only synthesize certain types of molecular components of proteins, much of the protein nutrition required for proper physiological functioning needs to come from the diet. Adequate amounts of proteins in the diet provide the various amino acids, building blocks of proteins and many structures in the body, to support proper growth and development. Some of these amino acids can be synthesized within the body but most are considered essential to the diet. In general, animal-based proteins provide the proper balance of these necessary amino acids and are considered to be of "higher quality" for this reason.[2] However, vegetarian sources of proteins can be equally beneficial. Since single plants may not contain the ideal ratio of various amino acids, it is important to combine different sources of vegetable-based proteins in the diet to achieve this balance. The common universal cultural practice of eating rice and beans together exemplifies this point: rice provides an amino acid, lysine, which beans lack.

While animal sources can provide the correct amino acid ratios, it is not recommended to excessively consume meats, dairy, and eggs in the diet. Instead, it is recommended to moderate the amount of animal-based proteins, which are associated with a variety of disease patterns such as cancer, heart disease, and obesity.[6] Vegetarian sources of high quality proteins include a variety of nuts, seeds, beans, and legumes. Even vegetables and fruits and whole grains contain small but necessary amounts of amino acids. The ideal range of proper protein intake varies from individual to individual based on activity levels, gender, age, and especially pregnancy and lactation status. It is best to consult a nutritionist or a physician trained in the field of nutrition to come up with the ideal protein quantity and foods in the diet. For most adults, a good range is 46 to 63 grams of protein daily. Excessive amounts of protein can increase the excretion of calcium in the urine.[7] In fact, high-protein diets, especially meat-based, which are very common in the United States, seem to be correlated to problems like osteoporosis. Diets excessively high in proteins are not recommended for anyone with impaired liver or kidney function[1] since they can be taxing to the digestive and urinary systems.

For individuals with CFS, the diet should consist of no more than 60 grams of protein daily for the average adult, except during pregnancy, lactation, and times of acute stress or injury. A general rule of thumb is to consume 10 to 20 grams of protein with each meal and to focus more on a variety of vegetarian sources of proteins such as beans, legumes, nuts, and seeds instead of animal sources. This provides adequate quantity and quality of proteins needed for energy, maintenance, and repair, while preventing the adverse consequences of a diet high in meats.

Fats

Fats are usually found in the forms of lipids, triglycerides, simple fatty acids, or cholesterols in the body. They comprise important components of cell membranes in virtually all cells of the body. They also make up most of the tissue found in the brain and the rest of the nervous system. In addition, fats can form more complex structures known as sterols, a category that includes cholesterol, steroid hormones, bile salts, and fat-soluble vitamins such as vitamins A, D, E, and K. Fats are the preferred storage form of energy, giving the body fuel reserves for energy needed at times of higher activity and reduced caloric intake. Fats provide protection around organs, insulation under the skin for maintaining body temperature, and transport mechanisms for certain nutrients in the body. When fats are consumed in the diet, they tend to improve the palatability of food, prolong the time that food stays in the stomach for better digestion and absorption, and provide the feeling of fullness and satisfaction (or satiety).

Like carbohydrates, fats have unfortunately received a bad rap from many fad diet plans. Not all fats are problematic, however. In fact, humans absolutely need certain types of fats for proper physiologic functioning. These fats are called "essential fatty acids" because they cannot be made in the body and are thus required through the diet. These are linoleic acid (omega-6 fatty acids) found in nuts and seeds such as safflower, sunflower, sesame, soy, corn, and others, and alpha-linolenic acid (omega-3 fatty acids) found mainly in most wild fish, wild game, and flax seeds. In addition, all dietary fats are divided into categories according to their level of saturation, or lack of double bonds in the molecular structure. Saturated fats, which do not have any double bonds, and trans fatty acids whose structures are changed chemically, are both implicated in cardiovascular and cancer-related health conditions.[8,9] Foods high in saturated fats include meats and dairy products, while foods high in trans fats include hydrogenated oils, margarine, vegetable shortening, and most processed foods made with these ingredients. Monounsaturated and polyunsaturated fats contain one (mono) or more (poly) double bonds and are found in olive oil, nuts, seeds, and even whole grains. These, along with omega-3 essential fatty acids, offer health benefits such as protection from heart disease, cancer, diabetes, and other chronic illness.[10,11,12]

For individuals with CFS, a diet that is low to moderate in fat intake is best. This means that about 15 to 30 percent of the total daily calories should come from fats. Even more important than the quantity of fats is the quality of fats. A diet rich in omega-3 essential fatty acids and mono- or polyunsaturated fats offers all the benefits of energy, vitamin storage, and hormonal and cognitive support, without the negative consequences of the trans fatty acids and saturated fats in terms of heart disease and cancer. Again, it is best to consult a health-care practitioner about nutrition for individualized dietary guidance before making drastic changes to the diet.

Water

Over two-thirds of the human body is made up of water alone. This amounts to an average of about 10 gallons of water in the adult human body.[1] Every function and process occurring in the body requires water as its very foundation; in fact every biochemical reaction of the body takes place in water as its solvent. Water plays a significant part in the normal processing of the digestive, urinary, cardiovascular, and lymphatic systems, to name just a few. It is also vital for maintaining proper body temperature. Water is necessary for all of the digestive organs to function and for nutrients in foods to be absorbed into the bloodstream. Because water comprises most of the volume of blood, it is the driving substance that enables nutrients to circulate through the blood vessels throughout the body. It also allows for waste products, toxins, and unnecessary chemicals to be expelled from the body. In addition, water makes up most of the lymphatic fluid that circulates immune cells throughout the body for protection and defense. The body cannot live more than a few days without water. And there are no substitutes for pure water either. Even mild dehydration, which is very common, can result in reduced physiological function and overall performance.[13]

The average adult requires about six to eight glasses, or 48 to 64 ounces, or up to 2 liters of water daily to prevent dehydration and slowing down of the various systems. A good way to measure individual needs for water is to divide total body weight (in pounds) by half to come up with the number of ounces of water required for daily consumption.

Ideally, water should be filtered to prevent contamination with heavy metals, microorganisms, and other unhealthy substances. Much of the U.S. water supply has been pumped with chlorine and fluorine for sanitation and dental reasons. But much of it is also contaminated with toxic compounds such as polychlorinated biphenyls (PCBs), pesticide residues, and nitrates, and heavy metals such as lead, mercury, and cadmium. A good quality water filter can remove most of these contaminants, making water safer for consumption.

MICRONUTRIENTS: VITAMINS AND MINERALS

Vitamin is the shortened version of the original name "vital amines." The term "vital" implies the level of necessity in the diet. Vitamins are substances that serve as cofactors to virtually all cellular functions and biochemical reactions in the body. Even though they fall under the category of micronutrients because they are needed in small amounts, they are still irreplaceable in terms of their contribution to healthy functioning. Many vitamins help with the digestion, metabolism, and absorption of nutrients in the body. They also play important roles in the cell's production of energy, as well as in the body's process of eliminating toxins and unwanted substances.

Minerals come from naturally occurring elements found in the earth. Like vitamins, they too act as cofactors for the body's multitude of cellular and biochemical processes. They build components of the blood, the way that iron incorporates into hemoglobin; they strengthen the musculoskeletal system, the way that calcium and magnesium deposit in bones; and they serve the body as electrolytes, the way that sodium and potassium excite nerve function. Some minerals, such as calcium, are needed in abundance for building structures of the body. Others fall into the category of trace minerals; even though they are needed in smaller amounts they are just as necessary.

Together, vitamins and minerals work synergistically to ensure ideal functioning in all the systems. These nutrients found in whole foods occur in their natural states, intermingled with macronutrients and enzymes to aid in their absorption and usage. Highest sources of vitamins and minerals are found in fresh fruits and vegetables and whole grains, which is why these foods are so important in the diet. Vitamins and minerals build enzymes, which catalyze numerous metabolic reactions in the body. They also comprise antioxidants, compounds that reduce the effects of free radical damage in the body, often referred to as oxidative stress.

Vibrant health and longevity can be attributed to the consumption of an abundance of these nutrients in the everyday diet. The Recommended Daily Allowances (RDA values) for these micronutrients were created to define the minimal amounts needed for overt disease prevention. However, these values tend to fall short of what most people require for optimal wellness. And, in the treatment of diseases, significantly higher doses are needed. Many of the nutrients needed for good health can be found in a healthful diet. But for most people, these levels are just not enough. A pure, high quality multinutrient formula is a good idea for individuals suffering from CFS, as well as for most individuals wanting to supplement their diets with a balanced formula. The best way to benefit from supplementation, above and beyond a good diet, is to consult a physician knowledgeable about nutrition to guide in nutritional treatment for this condition. In addition, many of these nutrients are spotlighted in the following chapter for their benefits in the treatment and support of CFS.

CAFFEINE AND SWEETENERS

Caffeine has become a popular part of the American culture, with people getting accustomed to regular use of this stimulant to fight off lethargy. It is found in coffee, black tea, chocolate, and most soft drinks. While caffeine can temporarily alleviate tiredness, its regular intake can actually worsen chronic fatigue. Momentarily, caffeine stimulates the brain to function better, enabling clarity of thoughts, increased work speed, and curbed drowsiness. After a short time, though, the original tiredness returns, and a person may need a higher dose of caffeine the next time to delay the inevitable lethargy.[14]

People with CFS face the same problem. In fact, regular use of caffeine as a stimulant tends to worsen chronic fatigue. A study of mice given a single dose of caffeine revealed improved swimming capacity.[15] But that same dose given consistently for 6 weeks led to an opposite effect, a significant reduction in their swimming capacity! Beyond the issue of reduced endurance, there seems to be a correlation between high caffeine consumption and psychiatric illness. A survey of psychiatric patients at a hospital showed that the degree of fatigue was directly proportional to the amount of caffeine consumed. The higher the amount of caffeine, the higher the fatigue reported.[16] Reducing caffeine intake slowly over a few days or weeks may help to avoid the withdrawal experienced by many who abruptly discontinue drinking coffee.

A similar pattern of quick energy followed by a more dramatic drop in energy occurs with simple sugar consumption. All concentrated sweeteners, including white and brown sugars, honey, maple syrup, molasses, barley malt, rice syrup, and fruit-juice sweeteners break down very quickly in the body and cause a rapid rise in blood sugar. A rapid rise in blood sugar provides only brief stints in energy, followed by a longer period of lethargy, inducing another craving for more sugar. Over time, the body becomes more and more fatigued with the blood sugar changes, and this can lead to a general sense of depletion. Since not much is known yet about the safety and long-term biochemical effects of artificial sweeteners, it is best to avoid them as much as possible.

GENERAL GUIDELINES FOR HEALTHFUL DIETARY HABITS

Eat a variety of fruits and vegetables to prevent chronic diseases. The overwhelming evidence in the medical and scientific literature as to the health benefits of plant-foods has led to a rise in the popularity of advocating for a diet high in these foods. A range of different fruits and vegetables will provide multitudes of vitamins, minerals, trace elements, enzymes, and antioxidants necessary for optimal health and prevention against disease. The plant-based compounds in fruits and vegetables are categorized as phytochemicals. These nourishing factors include fibers, enzymes, pigments such as carotenes, chlorophyll, and flavonoids, and antioxidants like vitamin C, vitamin E, and selenium.[17,18,19,20]

Consume whole grains rather than refined flour products. Refined sugars and white flour products cause a rapid rise in blood sugar, which the body responds to by releasing insulin. Eating a high-sugar diet over time causes tissues in the body to become insulin-resistant, leading to problems such as poor blood sugar regulation, obesity, and ultimately type II diabetes and heart disease.[21,22,23] Diets high in simple sugars and refined carbohydrates can promote the development of cancer and increases the risk of heart disease as well. Whole grains, which are full of fiber, B vitamins, and many other nutrients, lessen the rapid spike in blood sugar and thereby reduce the risk of these disease states.

Reduce the dependence on meat and animal-based foods. Increase vegetarian sources of proteins instead. The scientific evidence behind meat and animal product intake and the higher risks of heart disease and cancers is staggering. Diets higher in plant-based foods reduce the very risks associated with high animal intakes.[24,25] Meats contain cancer-causing compounds such as pesticide residues, heterocyclic amines, and polycyclic aromatic hydrocarbons, which form when meat is grilled, fried, or broiled.[26] In addition, meat and other animal products do not share the abundance of phytochemicals found in plant-based foods. Instead, meat contains higher levels of saturated fats, which are also implicated in many of the chronic diseases we face as national epidemics today.

Choose beneficial fats in the diet. Diets high in saturated fats and cholesterol are implicated in numerous cancers, leading the American Cancer Society and the National Cancer Institute to encourage less than 30 percent of calories from fat. It is important to maintain a diet enriched in omega-3 fatty acids and mono- or poly-unsaturated fats, while reducing omega-6 fatty acids, saturated fats, and trans fatty acids. The latter, which are found in margarine, shortening, and hydrogenated vegetable oils, disrupt cell membranes by making them less flexible than normal. Virtually every chronic disease can be traced back to the alteration in cell membrane function. As Drs. Murray and Pizzorno so aptly put it, "Without a healthy membrane, cells lose their ability to hold water, vital nutrients, and electrolytes. They also lose their ability to communicate with other cells and to be controlled by regulating hormones, including insulin."[1] On the other hand, diets high in monounsaturated fats and omega-3 fatty acids have the opposite protective effect.[8,9,10,11]

Limit the intake of food additives and pesticides. Studies show that farmers exposed to pesticides have higher risks of lymphomas, leukemias, and cancers of the stomach, prostate, brain, and skin.[27,28,29] Some chemicals such as DDE, DDT, PCB, pentachlorophenol (PCP), dieldrin, and chlordane can act like the hormone estrogen. Not only do these chemicals raise the risk of lymphomas, leukemia, and pancreatic cancer, but they also play a role in low sperm counts and reduced fertility in men.[30] Children aged 2 to 4 years eating organic fruits and vegetables had six times lower pesticide metabolites than those eating conventional produce! This recent University of Washington study[31] recommended avoiding foods with high pesticide residues, such as cantaloupes, green beans (canned or frozen), pears, strawberries, tomatoes (Mexican grown), apples, and winter squash. In addition to pesticides, many food additives have been linked to problems such as depression, asthma or other allergy, hyperactivity or learning disabilities in children, and migraine headaches.[32,33,34,35]

Eating Mindfully

It matters not just what we eat, but also how we eat. In our culture of fast foods, convenience, time restraints, and social isolation, meals seem to have become more of a hassle than an event to be relished. Many individuals perceive choosing foods and preparing meals as sources of stress and conflict and internal judgment. Rather, we can choose to perceive eating as a more joyous experience, one that is nurturing and fulfilling to the body, mind, and spirit. Reviewing the many psychosocial and spiritual aspects to food and eating goes beyond the purpose of this book. Instead, most meals can be improved dramatically just by slowing down and taking in the whole process to allow the body a chance to fully metabolize foods and assimilate all the nutrition. Here are a few reminders to help make meal time more enjoyable, and nutrition more absorbable.

- Take time to taste, smell, and look at foods. Chew thoroughly before swallowing, and take a moment before the next bite.
- Try to make meal preparation more enjoyable and less stressful by inviting creativity and play into the process. Consider listening to music in the background, using creativity to design a better presentation, bring family members or friends in to help with cooking or cleanup.
- Remember to eat sitting down whenever possible. The act of sitting helps bring the nervous system into a more relaxed state (parasympathetic dominance), which in turn allows the body to digest and absorb nutrients more effectively.

- Consider turning off or ignoring common distractions while eating such as traumatizing news flashes on television, ringing phones, and computer e-mail alerts.
- Going for a short stroll or amble after larger meals may aid in the digestive process and prevent the urge to overeat.
- Eat only when hungry, and stop once full. Overcome the obligation of "finishing the plate" by knowing that you can resume whenever you need to.
- Share meals with people who bring joy.
- Savor each bite thoroughly before the next one.

Fasting and Cleansing Diets

The art of fasting has been practiced for thousands of years by people in various cultures around the world. It is a philosophy and methodology designed to give rest to the digestive system, support liver detoxification pathways, and help the body eliminate unwanted buildup of wastes. There are many different techniques for fasting, each with its own merits and challenges, and each suitable for a particular personal constitution. While many disregard fasting or cleansing diets as starvation or food deprivation or punishment, in actuality these methods can offer therapeutic benefits when done correctly. Evidence supports the subjective improvements in emotional well-being and moods.[36] Fasting and cleansing diets are not suitable or ideal for everyone as they can create more harm than good if done inappropriately. So fasts and cleansing diets should only be done under the supervision of a licensed health-care professional with expertise in these practices.

There is potential benefit in fasting for those suffering from chronic fatigue and chronic disease in general. A study of 209 individuals with chronic pain and exhaustion syndromes underwent 7-day medically supervised fasts consisting of 250 calories and 3 liters of fluid daily. They reported a decrease in moods during days 3 and 4, with a subsequent improvement in both mood and sense of well-being. This study found no side effects to the fasting and concluded that it was a safe practice for those with chronic exhaustion and pain syndromes.[37]

A case study of one individual with CFS undergoing cognitive behavior therapy for treatment started experiencing anxiety about returning to work, causing his symptoms to return. Once started on a fasting treatment, he was considered to be "successfully rehabilitated."[38] The researchers suggested that the therapeutic fasting helped to recover his natural killer (NK) cell activity and acylcarnitine levels. While the patient briefly experienced increased physical and mental symptoms transiently during the fast, his self-confidence returned shortly afterward.

Another study on twenty-eight patients with chronic pain syndromes revealed why fasting might be so beneficial in long-term illness of this type.[39] The volunteers undergoing a 7-day fast of 300 calories per day demonstrated neuroendocrine activation. They experienced a rise in their cortisol levels, among other adrenal hormones, which was sustained for some time even after the fasting period was completed. This general activation of the HPA pathways induced by fasting might be clinically beneficial to individuals with CFS as well. Surprisingly, there was little complaint of hunger or chilliness, two side effects concerning many who choose to embark on some form of therapeutic fasting. Instead, there were very few side effects at all, and nearly all of the volunteers who fasted reported "great beneficial effect" and desire to participate in fasting again.

The Elimination Challenge Diet

As mentioned in an earlier chapter on etiologies, there is some evidence to support the connection between intensity of CFS symptoms and food intolerances. An intolerance is different from a food allergy in that the former invokes a more long-term subtle immune reaction. These reactions can manifest with symptoms such as digestive upset, fatigue, subtle mood and behavior fluctuations, joint inflammation and pain, all leading to chronic illness. Consumption of the problem foods induces release of cytokines in the bloodstream, an immune parameter whose levels are high in CFS. Several studies cited in the "Etiologies" chapter reveal the positive outcomes of CFS volunteers who reduced intake of some common food intolerances. These volunteers tried an elimination-challenge diet to experience relief in symptom severity while avoiding those foods.

So for many individuals who may not be able or willing to undergo a fasting or cleansing diet, an elimination-challenge diet may be the next best experience. Considered the gold standard for evaluating food intolerances and allergies, this diet involves first the elimination of suspected foods for 2–6 weeks. The most common foods to avoid at this time are wheat, dairy, corn, citrus, nuts, eggs, tomatoes, caffeine, alcohol, and soy. After the elimination of these foods, each food group is reintroduced one at a time into the diet. It is important to observe if any adverse reactions or flare-ups of symptoms occur during this experiment. Typically, these would be skin rashes, headaches, fatigue, mood changes, indigestion, bloating, constipation or diarrhea, symptoms involving the eyes, ears, nose, or throat, and any other symptoms characteristic of CFS. If within 24 hours of eating this particular food no symptoms occur, then the individual tries out another food category. If symptoms do occur, then the individual must wait until they resolve before experimenting with the next food group. This process continues until all suspected problem foods have been tried and tested.

In addition to serving as a tool for identifying possible food intolerances, the elimination-challenge diet offers the opportunity to try a more hypoallergenic diet, one free of most additives, preservatives, and other artificial ingredients. It also automatically encourages a higher consumption of whole foods and vegetables, which in and of itself is an improvement for most. Once food intolerances are identified, they should be avoided completely for about 2 months while the body becomes desensitized. Beyond that, the specific foods can generally be rotated into the diet about once or twice a week without causing flare-ups of symptoms.

While it is recommended to try an elimination-challenge diet with the guidance of a practitioner trained in this technique, this is a relatively basic experiment that can be done at home. To summarize the steps:

- Follow a hypoallergenic diet for at least 2 weeks by eliminating all foods containing wheat, dairy, corn, nuts, eggs, seafood, beef, potatoes, tomatoes, soy, bananas, citrus, refined sugar, alcohol, any artificial ingredients like MSG (monosodium glutamate), and all caffeine products like chocolate, tea, coffee, or soda.
- During the 2 weeks, make note of any symptoms arising out of "withdrawal" from these foods.
- After the 2 weeks of elimination, test out one food group at a time by eating it at each meal for 1–2 days. If a reaction occurs, record it, and wait until the symptoms clear completely before testing out the next food group.
- Once all the foods have been tested, try to avoid eating the problem foods for 1–2 months to give time for the immune system to desensitize.
- After a few months, the suspected foods can be enjoyed on occasion, rotating them within the diet no more than twice weekly.

EXERCISE AND MOVEMENT

Movement of the body is crucial to maintaining healthy functioning. Just about all forms of exercise, no matter how simple or gentle, can stimulate blood and lymphatic circulation, improve moods, balance the endocrine or hormonal pathways, maintain normal body weight, release natural endorphins or "feel-good" chemicals throughout the body, and enhance the immune system. Physical activity is a wonderful way to alleviate the effects of stress and strain from chronic illness.

For healthy people and people suffering from chronic illness, exercise can greatly improve the mood and mental outlook by reducing the negative effects of long-term stress on the body. In fact, regular exercise serves as a good coping method to encourage a better way of handling stress.[40] Exercise can also dramatically improve immune function by increasing (nearly doubling) the natural killer cell activity.[41,42] This provides a perfect benefit for those with CFS who deal with lowered immune cell activity at this level.

For many people, the word "exercise" often conjures up images of competitive rigorous activity to the point of exhaustion. But this level of intensity is not really necessary or even healthful for most people. In reality, intense athletic training can actually have opposite suppressive effects on the body's immune system.[43] Instead of "weekend warrior" workouts, it is more beneficial to embrace light to moderate activity on a daily basis. For example, it has been shown that gentle forms of exercise such as T'ai Chi are very effective for improving immune function.[44] T'ai chi is a type of martial arts that embraces flowing movement from one posture to another. As it is, most people with chronic fatigue may have a difficult time initiating any exercise regimen. Some may experience more than usual amounts of muscle pain and postexertional fatigue due to the chronic illness.[45] An ideal approach for them would be gentle light exercises on a regular basis, slowly working up to moderate activity.

Graded exercise therapy is a very useful tool in CFS. This type of routine recommends beginning with gradual walking and weight exercises, and later increasing time and intensity according to individual comfort and tolerance levels. This approach may be more helpful than just using flexibility and relaxation techniques alone.[46,47]

The importance of regular activity can be demonstrated by the fact that the *lack* of exercise induces symptoms common to CFS. In a study of eighteen healthy individuals who refrained from exercise for 1 week, eight of the volunteers reported a 10 percent increase in pain, fatigue, or depressed mood.[48] Laboratory testing discovered lower endocrine function measured as decreased cortisol levels, reduced immune function measured as reduced NK cell activity, and reduced autonomic function measured by heart rate variability. The authors suggested that some healthy individuals with a suboptimal stress response system tend to unknowingly exercise regularly to enhance better functioning of these systems.

COPING EMOTIONALLY

Any chronic disabling condition can leave an individual feeling challenged, anxious, or even hopeless. It seems understandable that someone dealing with CFS would experience anxiety, depression, and the nagging question of "Why me?" Mood and sense of well-being are tightly connected to energy levels and healthy functioning of the immune and neuroendocrine systems of the body. When energy levels are low, mood can be depressed, causing suppression of the immune system and imbalance of the hormonal pathways. These imbalances can further lead to lack of energy and diminished sense of vitality. A vicious cycle such as this is not uncommon in CFS and needs to be addressed for therapy to be comprehensive and complete.

Many people with CFS are aware, at least in part, of why they feel the way they do. In a qualitative interview with women suffering from CFS, the participants revealed that their lifestyle increased their vulnerability for this condition by reducing their resistance to stress.[49] The women interviewed in this study hypothesized that their immune systems were not as strong as that of their male counterparts, and that CFS was induced by a virus that they were more likely to catch because of this. In addition, they perceived that the emotional strain from pressures put upon them, or pressures they put upon themselves, also led to their increased vulnerability. Factors such as internal and external pressures, workload burdens, emotional conflict, and lack of relaxation were all gendered dimensions that may have reduced their resilience against these stressors. If this hypothesis can be extrapolated for most people with CFS, then the need for stress reduction, emotional support, and physical strengthening against the effects of stress is paramount.

There is a strong correlation between CFS and mental health issues such as anxiety and depression. One author recommends "pacing the energy" throughout the day to prevent complete burnout and flare-up of symptoms. Exercise and counseling using cognitive behavior therapy seem to be effective according to this writer.[50]

It probably does not help that so many CFS sufferers are told that their symptoms are "all in their head" or that "there is no cure" and it is something they "just have to live with." The lack of social support among caregivers, family members, friends, and especially healthcare providers to CFS sufferers can be mind-boggling, not to mention disheartening.[51] While it is important to maintain a positive mental outlook, it is unrealistic to expect that shift in perspective to magically occur on its own when the individual is dealing with the disability of CFS. Therefore, it is vital for healthcare providers and caregivers alike to convey the hope of improvement.

When interviewed, many individuals with CFS shared concerns over the lack of emotional support from their doctors.[52] In addition, they complained about the insufficient information given to them and about the confusion and disagreements over the causes of illness. One article best explained the role of the medical professional in all of this: "Doctors need to challenge their strong beliefs regarding medically unexplained conditions, where facts still remain unresolved. Recognizing this, the doctor may provide realistic support and advice, and contribute to the establishment of common ground for understanding and managing the condition."[49] Perhaps the best support a health-care provider can offer is empathy and understanding to an individual suffering from CFS. From a place of trust and rapport between doctor and patient, communication can begin about diagnostic testing, therapeutic options, and follow-up care. Just as important is the individual's desire and hope in achieving wellness through lifestyle changes, psychological support, natural medicines, and anything else needed for the evolution in their health.

Individuals suffering from CFS can experience great benefits from some basic lifestyle changes. Vitality in life comes from a diet filled with fresh vegetables and fruits, whole grains, nuts and seeds, good fats, and plenty of pure water. Detoxifying the body of metabolic waste products, including popular fixes such as sugar and caffeine, can be done with therapeutic medically supervised fasting and elimination-challenge diets. Combined with regular gentle activity and emotional support, these lifestyle changes support a healthy mind-body and lay the very groundwork for which other natural therapeutics may be effective.

CHAPTER 8

Nutrients

Well-rounded nutrition provides so much of the physical and biochemical nourishment to the body, allowing it to function normally and even optimally. In many diseases and conditions, deficiencies in nutrients are common culprits that should not be overlooked. In chronic fatigue syndrome (CFS), many of the characteristic symptoms overlap with those symptoms induced by chronic malnutrition. The medical literature points out that several specific nutritional deficiencies are part of the very etiology (cause) or pathophysiology (development) of CFS. In fact, marginal nutritional deficiencies not only contribute to the symptoms and clinical signs of the condition, but they also work against the body's inherent healing tendencies. Without nourishment and all of the factors necessary for normal physiology, the body functions start to deteriorate, leading to a state of disease and weakened ability to recover from that state. Once those nutrients are replenished, the body can begin to rejuvenate and normal physiology can resume.

The most common nutrient deficiencies found in the medical literature regarding CFS are antioxidants including vitamin C and Coenzyme Q10, several B vitamins, magnesium, zinc, essential fatty acids (EFAs), and amino acids such as L-carnitine. These are just a few that are currently being researched, but there are probably many more that have not yet been evaluated. While some of these nutrients can be tested for their concentrations and functionality, many cannot be readily evaluated. Usually, ruling out marginal nutrient deficiencies is difficult, expensive, and not always accurate due to many interfering factors.

To complicate matters, many individuals, despite having normal ranges of various nutrients upon testing, respond very well to treatment with those very same nutrients nonetheless. Clearly, their "normal" levels of nutrients do not seem relevant in lieu of using those nutrients in high doses as therapy. Therapeutic doses of nutrients confer almost pharmacologic effects in the body, correcting possible deficiencies and also promoting optimal functioning of physiology. Some of the therapeutic doses of vitamins and minerals may be hundreds of times higher than the daily recommended allowances, the latter being put in place just to prevent severe deficiencies that would cause pathology.

Many of the nutrients discussed in the following pages are safe enough for most people to use, even at their therapeutic ranges. And it seems reasonable for most individuals to support their overall health by supplementing with optimal dosages of multiple nutrients, easily done using a good quality multivitamin formula. However, as with true patient-centered practice of medicine, not everyone will respond the same way to each medicine. The holistic and alternative medical paradigm supports the idea of treating each person as a unique individual. So instead of passing out the same medication for everyone with the same condition, a safer and more effective approach would be to tailor or custom-design the therapy around the individual.

More often than not, medicines inherently found in nature from foods and medicinal plants can be very beneficial in supporting the body's ideal physiology as well as treating an individual with a specific medical condition. Serious adverse reactions to most vitamins and minerals are rare. However, remember that any and all "natural" substances can be extremely effective if used correctly and potentially harmful if used inappropriately. It would be best to consult a physician who is an expert in the field of nutrition and botanical medicines before embarking on a self-prescribed treatment regimen, not only to avoid possible problems with therapy but also to ensure the ideal amounts, dosages, timing, and types of treatment with nutritional supplementation from a place of clinical experience, scientific knowledge, and personal sense of intuition.

ANTIOXIDANTS

As mentioned in a previous chapter, CFS seems to be related to oxidative damage. When mitochondria (energy-producing structures in cells) start to dysfunction, free radicals or oxidants are generated. These free radicals produce serious damage to multiple organ systems and various tissues of the body, causing symptoms such as muscle pain and exercise fatigue. It is becoming clear that antioxidants are needed to reverse and prevent oxidative damage of CFS.

Researchers studied mice that were purposefully overworked to induce a state of chronic fatigue. They found that overwork caused oxidation of lipids and lowered levels of potent brain antioxidants such as superoxide dismutase and glutathione reductase. The treatment consisting of glutathione and herbal sources of antioxidants restored these levels, even better than administration of the commonly prescribed antidepressant Prozac![1] This is a clear example where natural treatments appear to be more effective than conventional protocol. In another experiment by the same group of researchers, mice were given botanical antioxidants, quercetin, and melatonin for treatment of artificially induced CFS. These treatments restored glutathione levels to their normal concentration and prevented lipid peroxidation.[2] The results of this study led its authors to suggest the use of antioxidants in treatment of CFS in humans as well.

Human studies have also shown that oxidative damage is related to CFS. In one experiment, thirty-three people with CFS had higher lipid peroxidation and increased susceptibility to cholesterol oxidation compared to people with just fatigue.[3] Oxidation of lipids and cholesterols is a general sign of oxidative damage, speeding up the aging process. The overall pro-oxidizing effects lead to long-term damage which relates to CFS symptoms. Since many antioxidants from natural sources have been known to reverse this damage, it seems obvious to use antioxidant therapy for treatment of people with CFS. In fact, an interesting study showed the synergistic effects of antioxidants for people with CFS.[4] An extract of Swedish pollen, containing multiple antioxidant nutrients and polyphenols, was given to twenty-two subjects with CFS over 3 months. One marker of oxidative stress, red blood cell membrane fragility, was remarkably improved in those who consumed the Swedish pollen. These same individuals also reported significant improvements in fatigue, sleep, digestive problems, and overall environmental hypersensitivity. While each nutrient played a role in this outcome, it was the synergy of them all that offered the most benefit.

Zinc

Zinc status has been found to be significantly lower in people with CFS compared to healthy individuals.[5] In fact, the lower the zinc status, the increased severity of CFS symptoms accompanied by increased subjective or personal experience of infection. A commonly used antioxidant that supports the immune system, zinc is correlated with T-lymphocyte activation. A zinc deficiency reduces the ability of CD8 T cells to function and links to signs of inflammation as well. When this particular type of T cell is impaired, the immune system lacks the ability to suppress excessive immune responses in general. Since CFS is characterized by excessive immune function overall, it is even more important for CD8 T cells to function in their modulating way. The authors of this study observed the lowered zinc status in individuals with CFS and encouraged zinc supplementation as one aspect of therapy.

In women with CFS, another study found red blood cell zinc concentrations to be significantly lower, even if the levels were within normal range, when compared to healthy volunteers.[6] In another study of 1,300 people with CFS, almost one-third had subtle zinc deficiencies.[7] While we know that zinc deficiency can lead to overall immunodeficiency,[8] it is interesting to note that low levels of this mineral can also cause fatigue and muscle pain.[9] Clinically, zinc is very useful as a dietary supplement for improving the function of the immune system, correcting possible deficiencies in people with CFS, as well as taming some of the symptoms of fatigue and muscle pain in these individuals.

Many antioxidants may be effective in treatment of CFS, as suggested by the authors of the study on Swedish pollen as a synergy of various antioxidants found in nature.[4] Currently, the clinical trials evaluating efficacy for each specific nutrient are few and far between. However, the following antioxidants have plenty of general clinical research to back up the idea of using them for treatment of CFS. Perhaps future studies will continue to show their usefulness.

Alpha Lipoic Acid

Alpha lipoic acid is a coenzyme vital for metabolizing sugars into energy in the form of adenosine triphosphate (ATP). As an antioxidant, it scavenges free radicals (products of oxidative damage).[10] It can also regenerate the body's own antioxidants, such as vitamin E, vitamin C, and glutathione.[11,12,13]

In the case of CFS, it provides protection to brain tissue against oxidative stress from metabolic dysfunction.[14] In a small trial of people infected with HIV, alpha lipoic acid improved blood antioxidant levels and improved the helper T lymphocyte ratios.[15] Even though this research was conducted on people with HIV, it may prove to be a promising option for people with CFS as well.

Glutathione and NAC

Glutathione is a potent antioxidant made in the liver. Its concentration reduces from binding up with and inactivating free radicals. Its supply is constantly in need of replenishing. Despite consumption of fruits and vegetables containing glutathione, it does not seem to be absorbed well in the gut.[16] Therapeutically, its precursor, N-acetyl cysteine (NAC), can be a more efficient way to replenish glutathione and reduce oxidative damage.[17]

In addition to being powerful antioxidants, NAC and glutathione increase helper T cell numbers and activity in people with HIV.[18] As mentioned earlier, although these results should not be forced to fit in with another condition, future research might find a similar immunological correlation with CFS.

Selenium

Selenium is a trace mineral found in vegetables such as broccoli, kale, onions, garlic, and other members of the Brassica plant family. It works by activating an enzyme called glutathione peroxidase,[19] which reduces oxidative stress by binding up free radicals and hydrogen peroxide.[20] Because of this action, selenium is often prescribed for people battling cancer for both treatment and prevention of recurrence. Selenium is often given with other antioxidants, such as vitamin E or vitamin C, because it tends to synergistically potentiate their effects.

Vitamin E

Vitamin E works closely with Vitamin C as an antioxidant, exerting therapeutic effects on organs such as the kidneys, the heart, the blood vessels, and even the brain.[21,22] In fact, Vitamin E also has an important role in supporting the immune system by enhancing the production and activity of natural killer cells (NK cells). This is an important part of the disease process in CFS, where individuals tend to produce ineffective NK cells. Interestingly, deficiency states generally affect the NK cell numbers and function in healthy people over age 90.[23] It makes good sense to use Vitamin E for the purpose of enhancing NK cell activity.

Vitamin C

Apart from its many diverse clinical uses and efficacy, Vitamin C is well known for its antioxidant and immune supportive properties. Its ability to change oxidative products into their neutral states marks its efficacy in oxidative stress conditions, such as CFS.[24] While this nutrient is readily available and abundant in most fruits and vegetables, subclinical deficiencies are more common in healthy people than recognized,[25] with the tendency to underdiagnose its depletion.[26] Interestingly, nonspecific fatigue and depression are the first symptoms of early depletion of Vitamin C.[27,28] Vague symptoms of fatigue, personality changes, and reduced motivation do in fact respond to supplementation.[29,30]

While it is not yet well-researched how vitamin C may affect those with CFS, it is well-documented that this nutrient enhances the immune system. Healthy people given 1 to 3 grams a day experienced improved circulation of a group of white blood cells called neutrophils toward viruses and bacteria that needed to be inactivated.[31,32] It also increased lymphocyte production and overall immunoglobulin levels.[33,34] And, Vitamin C's ability to activate the production of interferons and other immune mediators makes it beneficial in fighting viruses.[35]

All of these mechanisms for Vitamin C are valid and likely reliable in terms of clinical efficacy for CFS. However, there is yet another role that has been documented in the medical literature. Perhaps the most interesting connection between this vitamin and CFS is through the interactions of the immune system with the endocrine system. Immunologists have studied this connection well; immune cells have receptors for hormone signals, which either enhance or depress their ability to respond. Typically, glucocorticoids (such as cortisol) and androgens (such as testosterone) reduce immune cell reactivity while many other hormones (such as estrogens, insulin, and growth hormone) enhance immune function. Chronically elevated levels of glucocorticoids cause immunosuppression and result from prolonged bouts of stress induced by fear or anxiety, injury or pain.[36]

One study unraveled the relationship between vitamin C, immune status, and the endocrine system in CFS. The authors evaluated a man with CFS given an infusion of vitamin C with DHEA, a hormone from the adrenal cortex found to be in excess in those with CFS. This study found that the vitamin C infusion seemed effective at treating this person's CFS by activating his immune system to fight off infection. It also found that the vitamin C infusion produced a "rise in both insulin and cortisol by acting through the pituitary ACTH route," and that the physiologic enhancement of this vitamin on glucocorticoids was significant.

The authors supported a long-held theory that high concentrations of vitamin C in endocrine organs enhanced their hormone synthesis, and also that prolonged stress not only leads to elevated cortisol release but also to depression of vitamin C levels in the adrenal glands where this hormone is produced. They suggest that vitamin C infusions may help treat some people with CFS by "fortifying the activities of cortisol and testosterone."[37,38]

Magnesium

Magnesium, one of the most abundantly found minerals in the human body, is vital for proper functioning of many enzymatic reactions and chemical pathways. It remains central to the body's many metabolic processes. And without adequate amounts of magnesium, the body would have trouble getting many activities started in the first place. Currently, and historically, this mineral has been used to treat conditions such as anxiety, insomnia, organic mental disorders, muscle spasms and pain, and migraine headaches. Interestingly, magnesium deficiencies manifest very closely to those symptoms of CFS: weakness, fatigue, muscle pain and cramping, personality changes, and even learning disabilities. Research is finding that magnesium deficits are tied into CFS.

While oxidative stress is often blamed for causing age-related diseases, magnesium deficiencies may be just as pathogenic. In a study of ninety-three people with chronic fatigue, 54 percent of whom actually had CFS, a total of 47 percent also had magnesium deficiencies, which were not entirely caused by low dietary intake.[39] These individuals with magnesium deficit also suffered from a lower total antioxidant capacity. Oddly enough, even when supplemented with magnesium, many did not experience normalization of their total body magnesium stores. These same individuals also had persistently lower blood glutathione levels, suggesting a possible link between magnesium and the body's ability to reduce oxidative damage. Despite the inability to normalize total body stores, magnesium supplementation seemed to improve antioxidant capacity in general.

Improvement in antioxidant functioning might be why magnesium seems to improve symptoms of CFS. In one double blind placebo controlled clinical trial, those with CFS had a subtle but statistically significant lower red blood cell magnesium level than healthy controls.[39] A total of thirty-two individuals with CFS were given either intramuscular injections of magnesium sulfate or placebo daily for 6 weeks.[40] Of the fifteen receiving magnesium, twelve individuals with CFS reported significant improvement in energy, moods and emotional well-being, and reduced pain. More than half of those receiving magnesium reported complete resolution of fatigue! In contrast, the placebo group found only three of the seventeen individuals noticing any improvement at all. Of them, only one individual reported improved energy and no one reported complete elimination of fatigue.

This trial reflects what scientists have been figuring out for the past few decades about chronic fatigue in general. Magnesium supplementation reduces fatigue.

And although some benefited most from injectable magnesium, many others improved with oral supplementation of magnesium alone.[41] Several studies from the 1960s showed improvements in fatigue from oral supplements of magnesium at about 1 to 2 gram daily divided dosages. Treatment of equal amounts of magnesium and potassium aspartate caused relief of fatigue in 75 to 91 percent of nearly 3,000 individuals compared to 9 to 26 percent of those in the placebo group.[42] One study of healthy men enduring prolonged standardized physical exercise to the point of physical exhaustion found a significant increase in their maximal exercise capacity when given oral potassium-magnesium aspartate.[43] In another clinical trial an overwhelming 91 percent of seventy-one individuals with chronic fatigue experienced positive changes in energy levels when given potassium-magnesium aspartates.[44] These results were very similar to a study done with fifty-seven individuals complaining of fatigue who were treated with potassium and magnesium aspartates, 1 gram of each daily for 4 consecutive weeks. Again, a prominent proportion (86%) of these individuals reported feeling better and being able to cope with daily activities without fatigue.[45] In many of these studies, positive effects could be noted within 4 to 5 days, and the benefits lasted long after the ending of the treatment in 4 to 6 weeks, with little or no return of the original fatigue.

These results strongly emphasize the importance of magnesium in treatment of general fatigue as well as CFS. Some find maximal advantage in using intramuscular injections or intravenous (IV or into the vein) therapies in order to move magnesium directly into the bloodstream.[46] A Myers' cocktail is an example of one way of therapeutic dosing of magnesium, as well as many other minerals, vitamins, and even botanical preparations. Dr. John Myers pioneered this technique of injecting vitamins and minerals directly into the veins for direct and rapid absorption. Among the many conditions he treated using this therapeutic modality, chronic fatigue and pain were among the most successful. In fact, the author of this article paying tribute to Myers, Dr. Alan Gaby, reported dramatic benefits in some and general improvements in several other CFS patients receiving IV nutrient therapy. Many of his patients became progressively healthier with continued injections and some were able to continue recovering even after the treatments stopped.

While intramuscular or intravenous therapies may be efficacious for some, most would still benefit greatly from using oral magnesium supplementation. One research article found that oral supplementation of magnesium restored levels in those with magnesium deficiency.[47] In addition, certain forms of magnesium may be more bioavailable and better absorbed than others. Magnesium bound to aspartate or citrate tends to be absorbed more easily than when bound to insoluble salts such as chlorides, oxides, and carbonates.[48] Both aspartate and citrate happen to be "Krebs cycle intermediates" or compounds that feed into a pathway, which produces energy by breaking down glucose, fats, and proteins. So, in addition to the benefits derived from oral magnesium supplementation to correct deficiencies and to treat CFS, the binding agents aspartate and citrate also provide relief of fatigue.

Essential Fatty Acids

Essential fatty acids, EFAs, have earned their name because they cannot be synthesized in the human body. They are essential to the diet and therefore must be acquired from outside sources. Typically, EFAs are found in nuts and seed sources such as evening primrose oil and flax seed oil, which provide the omega-6 fatty acids, and also marine sources such as fish and microalgae, which provide omega-3 fatty acids. Both omega-3 and omega-6 fatty acids are considered to be the main categories of EFAs.

Clinically, EFAs serve a vital role in synthesizing molecules of phospholipids, providing structure to the outermost protective layer of cells (cell membranes). They allow for membrane fluidity, communication from one cell to another, and communication within each cell through a process called signal transduction. Both dietary intake as well as disease processes can have effects on the fatty acid content of cell membranes.[49] With a diet rich in EFAs, the cell membranes can freely achieve transmission of important chemical signals. However, without adequate intake of EFAs, the risk of intensity, severity, and character of many disease states increases. CFS is no exception. Research has studied mostly the use of omega-3 EFAs in the forms of eicosapentaenoic acid (EPA) and docosahexaenoic acid (DHA) for treatment of CFS.

EPA is a long-chain omega-3 polyunsaturated fatty acid that is found in marine mammals, oily fish, and commercially prepared fish liver oils. EPA's well-known anti-inflammatory effects are exerted when it competes with arachidonic acid in cyclooxygenase and lipoxygenase pathways.[50] Reducing these inflammatory chemicals in the body translates to alleviation of pain, fatigue, and many other physiological processes associated with chronic disease. Other positive health benefits of EPA include reducing triglycerides, and normalizing blood glucose and insulin levels, especially in those with diabetes.[51] EPA can also improve the ratio of the "good cholesterol" HDL (which stands for high-density lipoprotein) to the "bad cholesterol" LDL (which stands for low-density lipoprotein) by increasing HDL cholesterol by about 12 percent.[52] While LDL increases fat deposition into blood vessels, increasing the risks for cardiovascular disease, HDL delivers that fat back into the liver for breakdown or conversion. In addition, EPA has been found to be useful in the treatment of depression,[53] in reducing mortality associated with cardiovascular disease,[54] and overall in treating a variety of conditions related to high levels of inflammation in the body.[55]

EPA has a partner polyunsaturated fatty acid called DHA. DHA, another type of omega-3 fatty acid derived from fish and microalgae, has very similar chemical properties as EPA. Because the body can enzymatically convert this fatty acid into EPA,[56] DHA can also be beneficial in reducing inflammation due to chronic disease processes, lowering triglycerides and raising HDL cholesterol, and reducing risk of mortality from heart disease. In addition, DHA is present in breast milk and is also an important part of brain development during the third trimester of pregnancy as well as the first few months of life after birth.[57] Finally, DHA has been shown to make up of the gray matter tissue of the brain[58] and plays roles in structural developmental aspects such as neuronal synaptic membrane development.[59]

In CFS, the inadequate levels of essential fats EPA and DHA seem to be directly connected to severity of symptoms. This might partially be due to poor dietary intake but also due to improper metabolism or usage of these fatty acids. One study found lowered levels of DHA in people suffering from CFS, with higher levels of proinflammatory fatty acids such as oleic acid and palmitic acid, which increase inflammation.[60] Perhaps, oxidative stress creates higher levels of the latter as byproducts from damage. Another group of researchers found changes in the ratios of EFAs similar to that observed in an exaggerated response to excessive or prolonged stress.[61] This gives credit to the idea of chronic stress taking its toll on the body by creating burnout and vital exhaustion. These authors attribute the altered ratios of EFAs to derangement in their metabolism. In other words, dysfunction in the way the body uses, converts, and breaks down these fatty acids creates changes in EFA levels, which match the changes seen in stress overload.

One explanation for the variety of body systems affected in CFS comes from this idea of altered fatty acid metabolism. EFA metabolic dysfunction explains the inadequate or excessive responses in the immune system, the nervous system's reaction to prolonged stress, and the endocrine system's response to stress witnessed by changes in the hypothalamic-pituitary-adrenal axis. For example, the exaggerated activity of the immune system in producing increased numbers of certain immune cells contrasts with the lower numbers and activity of the NK cells produced. Another example would be that of the blunted release of pituitary hormone ACTH compared to the elevated levels of DHEA with reduced levels of cortisol produced in the adrenal gland. Both of these examples show evidence of simultaneous excessive and inadequate functioning of the immune and the neuroendocrine systems. Again, these changes may be due in part to the changes in metabolism of EFAs.

One hypothesis for the disruption of EFA balance may have to do with reaction from viral illness. Persistent viral infections seem to inhibit the enzyme necessary to activate EFAs from their precursor fatty acids (the delta 6 desaturase enzyme), which impairs the cell's ability for communication. It becomes a vicious cycle where a viral infection creates the imbalanced ratios of EFAs, preventing interferon production, which would otherwise help the body fight off the virus.[62]

Several clinical trials have shown the benefits of EFAs in the treatment of CFS. A small case series of twenty-nine people with CFS who were ill for an average of almost 6 years were given a dietary modification of increased intake of EFAs along with graded exercise and psychological support.[63] Within 3 months, twenty-seven of the twenty-nine participants experienced a 90 percent improvement and greater than two-thirds were fit enough for full-time work duties. In the following 16 months, most of the participants continued to enjoy even further progress. A study of a single individual with a 6-year history of unrelenting CFS showed marked clinical improvement in 6 to 8 weeks when treated with EFAs alone.[64]

An MRI done of the brain at 16 weeks of therapy found reduction of the size of the lateral ventricle of the brain, and area whose enlargement had been previously reported in individuals with CFS. A follow-up trial in a series of people with CFS treated with high doses of EPA confirmed symptomatic improvement starting in 8 weeks, continuing into 12 weeks and longer.[65] This trial also found similar cerebral changes from use of EPA.

Earlier, in a much larger study, sixty-three individuals who were ill with postviral fatigue syndrome (the former name for CFS) for 1 to 3 years were treated with a combination of EPA and DHA for 3 months.[66] Each day, the participants received eight capsules containing 35 mg of gammalinoleic acid and 17 mg of EPA per capsule, or a total of 136 mg of EPA daily. At just the 1 month mark, 74 percent of the group improved from their baseline values. After 3 months of treatment, 85 percent continued to improve in areas such as severe fatigue, muscle pain, and psychiatric problems. These results were vastly different from those of the placebo group who regressed to their original state of condition. Laboratory testing revealed that participants had abnormally low levels of EFAs, which normalized with treatment. Also, the previously elevated monounsaturated and saturated fatty acid levels returned to normal range, demonstrating EFA's role in reducing proinflammatory fatty acid levels. The authors found no adverse effects from the therapy and concluded that the use of EFAs for treatment of CFS was "rational, safe, and effective."

Reduced levels of omega-3 fatty acids in twenty-two individuals with CFS were directly related to illness severity, pain, fatigue, and failing memory.[67] Not surprisingly, illness severity was correlated to higher levels of the more inflammatory fats such as omega-9, arachidonic acid, and saturated fats. The researchers made an interesting observation about the lower levels of EFAs. Reduced EFAs corresponded to decreases in blood zinc levels as well as decreased activation of T lymphocytes! This leads us to wonder if omega-3 deficiencies contribute to the pathophysiology of CFS through the immune system. This ties together the aspects of EFA imbalances, zinc deficiencies, and immune dysfunction.

The role of EFAs in treatment of CFS is apparent—those with CFS tend to have lower ratios of omega-3 fatty acids, their symptoms improve dramatically with EFA therapy in as little as several weeks, and treatment corrects the original deficiencies allowing for continued future progress. Adequate levels of EFAs also seem to prevent proinflammatory fatty acid elevations, reducing pain, fatigue, and other disease processes. And finally, there is a connection between omega-3 fatty acids, antioxidant status with zinc, and proper immune functioning in individuals with CFS. Clinical research strongly points to the need to supplement EFAs into the diet of those suffering from this condition.

THE B-COMPLEX VITAMINS: FOLIC ACID, VITAMIN B_{12}, AND NIACIN

Vitamin B complex refers to the essential water-soluble nutrients including thiamine (vitamin B_1), riboflavin (B_2), niacin (B_3), pantothenic acid (B_5), pyridoxine (B_6), biotin, folic acid, and the cobalamins (B_{12}). Even though these vitamins have been grouped together due to their sequential discoveries in extracts of rice, yeast, or liver, these nutrients do not really share much of a relationship to each other. However, each of the B vitamins has unique and specific functions in the body. Vitamins in general serve as cofactors to make enzymes work more efficiently. The various B vitamins help with producing energy and breaking down substances, support metabolism of nutrients and waste products, and promote cell division and maturation. Many people take Vitamin B complex regularly to combat the effects of stress, to acquire better energy and stamina, and to treat specific health conditions related to deficiencies of these nutrients. Several of the B vitamins may be useful, and even necessary, in treating CFS.

Folic Acid

Folic acid, also called folate, gets its name from the same source as the word "foliage" for green leafy plants. This is because this B vitamin is found abundantly in green leafy vegetables, such as spinach, kale, chard, broccoli, dark lettuce, and so on. Other foods that are naturally high in folate include okra, asparagus, most fruits, beans, mushrooms, and some animal proteins like beef liver.[68,69] Clinically, folic acid is vital for the synthesis of DNA, making it a requirement for proper cell growth and division into new cells. In addition, folic acid is a necessary nutrient during the development of the nervous system in as much as its deficiency in pregnancy can lead to neural tube defects.[70] One of the other benefits of folic acid is that it can reduce levels of homocysteine, an amino acid, which if elevated is a risk factor for atherosclerosis, thromboembolism, ischemic strokes, heart attack, and other cardiovascular diseases.[71] And, very pertinent to CFS, adequate amounts of folic acid relieves the effects of oxidative stress which seems to be part of the problem in this unique condition.[72]

There is a long history of folate deficiency that relates to chronic fatigue. In fact, folic acid has been commonly used to treat fatigue. For example, in one study of people experiencing easy fatigability with minor cognitive issues, taking folic acid supplements of at least 10 mg daily for 3 months started resolving their symptoms.[73] Folate deficiency overlaps with symptoms of CFS in that both share elements of fatigue, depression, and immune system dysfunction.[74] Perhaps folate deficiency contributes to the pathological development of CFS.

In order to address this idea, one study evaluated the proportions of those with CFS who actually had a folic acid deficiency. Out of sixty individuals with CFS, half of them had folic acid deficiencies, and an additional 13 percent were found to have low borderline concentrations.[75] Chronically low levels of serum folic acid correlate to low levels in the cerebrospinal fluid, a substance that bathes and nourishes the brain. According to one alternative medicine review article, this folate deficiency in the brain may cause cognitive impairment, leading to depression and other neurological deficits common to CFS.[76] While the research has yet to determine how treatment with folic acid might help those with CFS, long-term regular supplementation with folic acid seems to be very useful in the author's clinical practice.

Vitamin B$_{12}$

Vitamin B$_{12}$, also called hydroxyl-, methyl-, or cyano-cobalamin, has a close relationship to folic acid. Like folic acid, B$_{12}$ is responsible for maintaining normal growth and division of cells, and synthesizing DNA. Vital to cell reproduction and maturation, it supports healthy red blood cell development. It also helps synthesize myelin, a fatty sheath surrounding and protecting nervous tissues, making it important for rapid transmission of nervous signals in the brain and throughout the body. As a vitamin, B$_{12}$ serves as a cofactor or coenzyme to many metabolic processes. Along with folic acid, it converts homocysteine (a risk factor for cardiovascular disease) into methionine (an amino acid which does not pose such harmful risks).[77] Vitamin B$_{12}$ helps enzymes to breakdown fats and carbohydrates for use as energy sources, in addition to helping the body build more proteins for all sorts of physiological functions.

Unlike folic acid, though, this nutrient is not as readily available in fruits and vegetables. Instead, naturally occurring B$_{12}$ is created by microorganisms that thrive in the body's large intestine or colon. It can be found in animal sources such as meats, fish, and liver in the form of adenosylcobalamin and methylcobalamin. Cyanocobalamin and hydroxycobalamin are synthetic forms of vitamin B$_{12}$. The body requires a protein (called intrinsic factor) made in the stomach and activated by the gastric acids to absorb this vitamin in the intestines. Any substance interfering with stomach acid production and intrinsic factor synthesis can reduce absorption of B$_{12}$ leading to a condition called pernicious anemia. This B$_{12}$ deficiency condition is characterized by fatigue, depression, and weakness, very similar to those symptoms in CFS.

So how does vitamin B$_{12}$ relate to CFS anyway? It turns out that those with CFS may have higher breakdown of this vitamin. A study of over one hundred people with CFS showed elevated metabolite excretion revealing an overall vitamin B$_{12}$ deficiency state.[78] Again, the B$_{12}$ deficiency resembles the symptoms of fatigue and depression witnessed in CFS. Another study found that lower methylcobalamin levels in twelve women diagnosed with both CFS and fibromyalgia were linked to fatigability and neurasthenia.[79] This B$_{12}$ deficiency was directly related to elevated homocysteine levels, which were found in these participants. A possible conclusion is that those with CFS concomitant with fibromyalgia seem to share high levels of homocysteine in the central nervous system.

Just like with folic acid, there is a long history of using vitamin B$_{12}$ for treatment of unexplainable fatigue. A group of individuals suffering from chronic tiredness with no organic cause of disease experienced significant improvement in feelings of well-being when treated with B$_{12}$.[80] They were given 5,000 mcg of B$_{12}$ by intramuscular injections twice daily for 2 weeks. And interestingly, even though all the participants had normal serum B$_{12}$ levels, they all still benefited from treatment with this vitamin. The positive benefits lasted for at least 4 weeks even after the final administration.

These results were confirmed in another trial of fatigued individuals with normal B$_{12}$ concentrations.[81] Overall, those given the B$_{12}$ injections reported feeling better, with the maximum sensation of wellness resulting from substantial dosages, ranging from 3,000 mcg four times weekly to 9,000 mcg daily!

For therapeutic results, the dose of B_{12} needed to adequately treat CFS is massive compared to the recommended daily allowance, which is a mere 2.4 mcg daily. The RDA values are merely set in place to prevent and treat frank nutrient deficiencies, not to address a chronic illness. These massive doses can best be achieved through intramuscular or intravenous injections of 1,000 mcg weekly.[76] According to this regimen, once an initial response is achieved, the same dose can be administered less frequently—once monthly for as long as necessary.

Case in point, when treating 2,000 individuals with CFS, the use of 1,000 mcg of B_{12} daily got inconsistent results.[82] But when the clinicians increased the dosage to 2,500 to 5,000 mcg cyanocobalamin every 2 to 3 days, 50 to 80 percent of the participants responded with increased energy, stamina, and sense of well-being within a few weeks of commencing therapy. By contrast, another double-blind crossover study using both folic acid and vitamin B_{12} supplementation failed to report positive results.[83] This is most likely due to the smaller amounts being used; the researchers used 200 mcg of cyanocobalamin instead of 2,500 to 5,000 mcg in the previous studies.

One can conclude from these trials that the dosages necessary to achieve symptomatic improvement were substantially higher than the bare minimal levels needed to prevent a frank deficiency of this vitamin. One reviewer suggested that this must be due to an almost pharmacologic effect created by cyanocobalamin.[76] In other research reviewed by him, daily 5,000 to 10,000 mcg injections of B_{12} have been shown to induce analgesic effects, relieving pain in people with degenerative neuropathies, cancer, and vertebral pain syndromes.

There are some fascinating theories to explain Vitamin B_{12}'s therapeutic effects on CFS. One theory offers that in people with CFS, 40 to 100 percent of their red blood cells are "grossly deformed" or abnormally shaped.[84,85,86] The resulting rigidity and dimpling keep these red blood cells from being able to bend and fit into smaller blood vessels. When blood cannot freely flow through the microcirculation, the tissues and organs downstream end up being deprived of oxygen and nutrients, while toxic byproducts of cellular function accumulate in those areas.[87] One proponent of this theory suggests that this may be why people with CFS suffer from symptoms across multiple organ systems.

The use of vitamin B_{12} can correct the abnormal shape and structure of red blood cells. An open trial of people diagnosed with myalgic encephalomyelitis showed that they had higher proportions of abnormally shaped RBCs.[88] About half of those given 1,000 mcg of vitamin B_{12} intramuscular injections daily experienced improved sense of well-being within 24 hours. They also showed reduction in their proportions of deformed RBCs, whereas the other half who did not improve had no change in their RBC configuration. Again, this provides evidence to the idea that adequate dosages of B_{12} improved symptoms of CFS by normalizing red blood cell shape, allowing for better circulation into tissues.

Niacin, NADH, and Other B-complex Vitamins

Several other B-complex vitamins have been found to be deficient in those with CFS, namely riboflavin, thiamine, and pyridoxine.[89,90] While there are no clinical trials yet of the benefits of using these B vitamins for treatment of those with CFS, it may be beneficial to correct the deficiencies at the very least, and perhaps study the use of B-complex vitamins for actual symptomatic improvement.

Niacin, or vitamin B₃, is commonly used for lowering cholesterol and high blood pressure, as well as improving blood glucose regulation in people with diabetes and insulin-resistant conditions. Niacin is also known as niacinamide, nicotinamide, and nicotinic acid, even though each is a slightly different chemical variation from the other, and each has its own specific actions in the body as well. Vitamin B₃ is present in many foods including yeast, meat, fish, milk, eggs, green vegetables, and cereal grains.

Niacin and niacinamide are precursors of nicotinamide adenine dinucleotide (NAD) and nicotinamide adenine dinucleotide phosphate (NADP), which are essential for oxidation-reduction reactions, ATP synthesis, and ADP-ribose transfer reactions.[91] In other words, niacin gets converted into a substance called NAD, which helps the body make energy and supports many different types of reactions. During a deficiency of this nutrient, an individual might suffer from dermatitis (skin inflammation), diarrhea, and eventually dementia. This triad of symptoms from niacin deficiency is called pellagra, and is increasingly rare in industrialized nations due to the fortification of foods with vitamin B₃. While pellagra is not very common, subtle or subclinical deficiencies of many B vitamins are quite common since these nutrients become easily depleted with the use of various medications and poor dietary choices.

The use of niacin for various cardiovascular diseases is more and more popular. At merely 1 gram daily, vitamin B₃ can decrease total cholesterol by 8 to 21 percent and triglycerides and harmful cholesterol by 8 to 50 percent, while simultaneously raising HDL (the cardioprotective cholesterol) by 15 to 35 percent.[92] As another protective role against morbidity from heart disease, this nutrient reduces fibrinogen concentrations by stimulating its breakdown.[93] This slows down the clotting tendencies of slow-moving blood through areas of plaque formation in the blood vessels, reducing the chances for heart attacks and strokes to occur. A beneficial effect of niacin in the form of NADH (nicotinamide adenine dinucleotide, the active coenzyme form of vitamin B₃) is in countering the negative effects of jet lag on cognition and wakefulness.[94]

In CFS, niacin seems to provide improvement in quality of life. A double-blind study of twenty-six individuals with CFS received either 10 mg of NADH or placebo daily for 1 month.[95] After a washout period with no supplementation for 1 month, the participants were crossed into the opposite group for another 1 month of either treatment or placebo. A total of eight out of the twenty-six (31%) responded favorably, compared to only two (8%) in the placebo group. As no adverse effects were found, the authors concluded that this might be an effective therapy, and that a larger cohort study should be done in the future.

In another small trial, thirty-one individuals with CFS were treated with either NADH or psychotherapy for 24 months.[96] Their progress was closely monitored with questionnaires, physical examination, and a medical history every 3 months. The twelve patients who had received NADH experienced a dramatic and significant reduction in their symptom scores in the first part of the therapy. Subsequently, there did not seem to be much difference in the treatment groups after the first part. The authors concluded that a larger study needs to be done to further evaluate this discrepancy. Nonetheless, niacin seems to have an observable and considerable benefit in improving overall sense of wellness in those with CFS.

L-CARNITINE

An amino acid called L-Carnitine is found naturally in the body but is especially concentrated in cardiac and skeletal muscle tissues. This is because its function is to aid cells in producing energy. In fact, L-carnitine acts as an enzyme, which transports fatty acids into mitochondria, where these fatty acids get broken down to produce energy stored as ATP. Aside from its natural production in the human body, it can also be acquired in the diet from meat and dairy products, or synthesized from the amino acids lysine and methionine.

In addition to providing energy, L-carnitine has antioxidant properties.[97] In fact, another form of L-carnitine called acetyl-L-carnitine reduces chemicals of oxidative stress and prevents oxidative damage in the brain.[98] As carnitine is vital to proper muscular function, a deficiency often presents with skeletal muscle weakness, muscular dystrophy, damage to the heart muscles, irregular heart rhythms, and rapid lowering of blood sugar levels.[99,100] Therapeutically, this amino acid has been used to improve exercise performance, reduce muscle cramps and hypotension, and even to improve red blood cell survival in people undergoing dialysis.[101,102,103] Early research is showing carnitine to be effective for people with HIV in reducing the death of T-lymphocytes, namely CD4 and CD8 cells, thus improving their immune cell numbers overall.[104,105]

Several studies point to deficiencies in L-carnitine in people with CFS. One evaluation of thirty-five individuals with CFS found statistically significantly lower serum total carnitine levels.[106] The lower levels corresponded to increased symptom severity, while higher levels seemed to suggest improved overall functional capacity. Another study confirmed these results of lowered carnitine levels in those with CFS.[107] These researchers previously observed that a carnitine deficiency created an energy deficit or mitochondrial dysfunction in the mitochondria, explaining the CFS characteristic symptoms of fatigue, muscle pain and weakness, and postexercise tiredness.[108] They also found that with recovery of fatigue, the serum concentrations of this amino acid tended to increase. They propose using measurements of carnitine as one diagnostic tool and as a way to assess the level of severity or improvement in those with CFS.

Another group supported the idea of carnitine deficiency being related to mitochondrial dysfunction. They initiated a clinical trial comparing the effects of L-carnitine with amantadine, a pharmaceutical drug commonly used to treat fatigue in neurological conditions such as multiple sclerosis.[106] A group of thirty individuals with CFS were either given L-carnitine or amantadine for 2 months, with a 2-week washout time, followed by another 2 months of treatment using the opposite medication. More than half of the group given amantadine dropped out of the study due to the medication's side effects. Unfortunately, even those who managed to tolerate the medication did not benefit from a significant change in their clinical symptoms.

Interestingly, the group treated using 1 gram three to four times daily of oral L-carnitine found statistically significant improvement in twelve of the eighteen symptom parameters, with no deterioration in any at all. The authors concluded that L-carnitine was a very well tolerated medicine (with obviously fewer adverse reactions compared to amantadine) which improved clinical status in those with CFS in just about 1 month of treatment. This study boasts a terrific example of a natural medicine supporting clinical improvement in a condition for which drug therapy is ineffective and poorly tolerated. It seems that some benefited more dramatically than others. In fact, those who benefited from L-carnitine supplementation returned to normal functioning from a state of complete disability. This dramatic shift did not seem to be related to baseline levels of carnitine to start with, so there is no obvious predictor for those who will respond to supplementation this way.

COENZYME Q10

Coenzyme Q10 is a ubiquitous transporter of molecules involved in cellular respiration, a process by which cells make energy. Like L-carnitine and others, it works within mitochondria, the cell's energy-producing machines, and so abnormalities with CoQ10 may be indicative of mitochondrial dysfunction. Because CoQ10 is made in the body, it is not considered essential to the diet but can be taken in from meats and seafood. For achieving therapeutic range, supplementation of CoQ10 in the diet is required.

In addition to serving in the production of ATP for cellular energy, CoQ10 acts as an antioxidant, a stabilizer for cell membranes, and as a cofactor in many metabolic pathways.[42,109] Clinically, CoQ10 has been used to improve exercise tolerance.[110,111,112] This coenzyme is also used in conditions of deficiency such as congestive heart failure (CHF), hypertension, periodontal disease, certain muscular diseases, and AIDS.[42] With these conditions, the mechanism of action is that CoQ10 prevents oxidative damage, reduces free radical formation, increases ATP synthesis, and stabilizes cell membrane.[113] In fact, coenzyme Q-10 and L-carnitine work synergistically together to support mitochondrial energy production in cells, while protecting against oxidative and toxin-induced damage.[114,115]

This coenzyme has a dual purpose in those with CFS. It can serve as an antioxidant, replenishing concentrations of Vitamin E and Vitamin C during reduction of oxidative stress.[116] Coenzyme Q10 is also used primarily for its ability to improve mitochondrial function in the case of CFS.[117] Dramatic effects were observed in a study of twenty female participants with postexercise fatigue.[76] These individuals were so depleted that they needed bed rest following even mild forms of exercise. At baseline, 80 percent of them were found to have CoQ10 deficiencies, and these deficiencies worsened throughout the course of the day with normal activity and following exercise. After 3 months of CoQ10 supplementation at a moderate dose of 100 mg daily, their exercise tolerance more than doubled in every one of them. Almost all of them (90%) had either reduction or complete resolution of their clinical symptoms, and nearly the same number had reduced fatigue after exercise. While it will be even more confirming to see a clinical trial on people with CFS given CoQ10, this study alone gives a lot of credit to the idea of supplementing with CoQ10 to improve postexertional fatigue and mitochondrial function.

LACTIC ACID BACTERIA AND PROBIOTICS

The human body harbors many multitudes of thriving microorganisms. Some may be pathogenic and infectious. But the majority live symbiotically, feeding the cells of the intestines, helping the body absorb nutrients by releasing them from hard-to-digest foods, stabilizing an internal environment with the appropriate pH, and preventing growth of abnormal bacteria and fungi from inhabiting the digestive, urinary, and reproductive systems.[118,119,120,121] One of the most common types of this beneficial microbial flora is a category of lactic acid bacteria, commonly known as Lactobacillus species, obviously named for their ability to produce lactic acid in the gut. Some members of this group include *Lactobacillus acidophilus, L. bulgaricus, L. casei* sp. *rhamnosus, L. delbrueckii, L. fermentum, L. plantarum, L. reuteri, L. rhamnosus,* and *L. sporogenes.* Of these, *L. reuteri* is the most commonly occurring species in the gastrointestinal tract and in breast milk.[122] Aside from breast milk, these beneficial bacteria are found in fermented foods such as yogurt, sauerkraut, kim chee, as well as supplementally in powdered form or capsules. Historically and currently, the primary clinical uses of Lactobacillus have to do with preventing colonization of unhealthy bacteria and other pathogens during antibiotic therapy. Lactobacillus seems to prevent some of the side effects of antibiotic therapy, such as bloating, cramping, diarrhea, and overgrowth of fungi, just to name a few. If the beneficial bacteria is replenished during destruction of all the bacteria with antibiotics, then chance for secondary infection by harmful microorganisms is reduced.[123,124]

The human body relies on lactic acid bacteria for support in metabolizing foods (and drugs and chemicals), while also helping to synthesize and absorb nutrients such as vitamins and minerals, by making them more bioavailable.[125,126] These bacteria also reduce chances for permeability of substances in-between the intestinal cells by strengthening the intestinal barrier, thereby reducing risk and progression of atopic conditions such as allergies and asthma.[127,128,129] In addition, these friendly bacteria have impressive effects on the immune system by promoting its activity.[130,131] The overall effect is to increase activity of cytokines, lymphocytes, and reduce the part of the immune system that leads to allergies. *L. acidophilus* and *casei* have both been found to promote the production of EFAs in the human intestines.[132] And finally, research is beginning to show the very important antioxidant affects from *L. acidophilus* as well as *Bifidobacterium longum*.[133] Because of the multiple therapeutic effects of these bacteria and their ability to counteract the effects of antibiotic medications, they are commonly referred to as "probiotics."

One CFS expert has been studying these various beneficial effects of probiotics and their potential use in CFS.[134] It turns out that those with CFS tend to have "marked alterations in microbial flora," including lowered levels of Bifidobacterium species as well as small intestinal bacterial overgrowth. In the last few years, it is becoming understood from research that individuals with CFS tend to have more of an allergic profile, nutrient deficiencies or malabsorptions, and increased oxidative damage related to dysfunctions of their EFA levels. It seems that the inadequate levels of beneficial bacteria may be playing a part in the development of the nutrient deficiencies, fatty acid imbalances, and atopic or allergic tendencies. Lactic acid bacteria can influence the immune system function by inducing the helper-T cell response and controlling the allergic aspect of the immune system. This group of bacteria can also support synthesis of EFAs and enable better nutrient absorption in the intestines by reducing permeability and inflammation. And finally, lactic acid bacteria can work as antioxidants to reduce the levels of oxidative stress characteristic of CFS. Perhaps therapeutic administration of these probiotics would help to reduce the severity and disease progression with CFS. Typical doses are at least 10^9 numbers of viable bacteria per dose for each strain of Lactobacillus.[135] Future clinical trials will have to show exactly how these physiological benefits would manifest as symptom resolution and healing for this condition.

SUMMARY OF NUTRIENTS FOR CFS

Ideally, most of our nutrition should come from a diet rich in nourishing foods. A wholesome diet usually supplies a bounty of the vitamins, minerals, and other nutrients necessary to prevent diseases caused by frank nutritional deficiencies. Many, however, still develop marginal nutritional deficiencies from an imbalanced diet or from improper absorption or from disease process and medication use. In the long run, these minor deficiencies manifest with symptoms similar to CFS: fatigue, muscle pain and weakness, digestive disorders, immune suppression, and mental-emotional disorders. For individuals with CFS, much of the "disease process" can be affected by improving nutrient status. Table 8.1 outlines the most important, and best-researched, nutrients for treatment of CFS. A basic start would be to take a good quality multinutrient formula daily with meals, just to boost the amount of nutrients available for absorption into the system. In addition, it may also be wise to supplement the diet with an antioxidant formula, a vitamin B complex, fish oil or flax seed oil, and an everyday probiotic

Table 8.1. Nutrients for CFS

Nutrients	Dosages	Benefits in CFS
	B Vitamins	
Folic acid	800 mcg up to 10 mg daily if given by injection or intravenously for 3 months	Alleviates fatigue and depression. Always use in conjunction with vitamin B_{12} to prevent undiagnosed pernicious anemia!
Vitamin B_{12}	2,500 to 5,000 mcg by injection or intravenously twice weekly for 4 to 8 weeks	Alleviates fatigue, depression, and pain. Always use in conjunction with folic acid to prevent undiagnosed pernicious anemia!
NADH, niacin	5–20 mg daily	Enhances cellular energy production
	Antioxidants	
Vitamin C	1–2 grams daily (up to 10 grams if given intravenously)	Improves immune function
Glutathione	600 mg intravenously on alternate days for 2 months	Powerful antioxidant to reduce oxidative stress, general immune support
Alpha lipoic acid	300–600 mg daily	Antioxidant protection, nerve regeneration
Selenium	100–200 mcg daily	Restores immune function, supports synthesis of glutathione, enhances natural killer cell activity
Vitamin E	400–1200 IU daily	Antioxidant protection, nerve regeneration, stabilizes cell membranes, supports immune response
	Minerals	
Magnesium (aspartate or citrate or malate)	500–1,000 mg daily	Alleviates muscle pain, reduces fatigue
Zinc	30 mg daily, up to twice a day	Enhances antioxidant protection, supports muscle strength and endurance
	Other Nutrients	
L-carnitine	1–2 grams daily, up to three times daily for 3 months	Supports muscle strength and reduces fatigue

(Continued)

Table 8.1. *(Continued)*

Nutrients	Dosages	Benefits in CFS
Coenzyme Q 10	100 mg daily	Supports muscle strength and endurance, enhances cellular energy production
Essential fatty acids	1,000 mg DHA + EPA daily, or evening primrose oil 3–6 grams daily	Reduces fatigue and inflammation
L. *acidophilus*	10^9 viable bacteria per dose	Reduce allergies, improves nutrient absorption, and immune modulation

formula. In many cases, the best way to get therapeutic dosages of these nutrients is through an intravenous nutrient formula, designed specifically to target the needs of the individual. Since most CFS sufferers will require more than just a daily multivitamin, working with a holistic health-care practitioner can help to tailor a treatment plan to optimize wellness for each individual.

CHAPTER 9

Botanical Medicines

INTRODUCTION

Botanical medicines have been used all over the world in every different traditional medical culture. Virtually each plant has a myriad of medicinal and biochemical properties, whether or not human beings have figured them out. Research into plant-based medicines has been growing exponentially, especially with the increase in everyday usage in the United States. With each research study, we learn more and more about botanical medicines, helping to understand the best uses for these herbs in treating people with various clinical conditions. Case in point, the use of herbal medicines in treating chronic fatigue syndrome (CFS) is on the verge of taking off in the scientific literature. Beyond the research, though, there is a deep appreciative history of knowing how these plants benefit human health and wellness, passed on from thousands of years of clinical experience, anecdotal stories, legends, folklore, grandmother's home remedies, and the wisdom from trained healers like physicians, herbalists, shamans, and medicine women across the world.

The brilliance of botanical medicines is that each and every healing plant represents a panacea of medicinal properties. A given plant may offer dozens of clinical uses, depending on the part of the plant, the location and environment where it is grown and harvested, the careful process by which it has been prepared, and the knowledge and wisdom by which it is administered. Also, each plant contains chemicals, nutrients, plant-based hormones, and countless other compounds that work synergistically to generate its wealth of medicinal values. And because each constituent is found alongside another, potential adverse effects of any one constituent may be softened or even nullified by the properties of the other constituents. This is perhaps one of the clearest advantages of using botanical medicines over pharmaceutical-grade isolated chemical-based medicines. Plant medicines tend to be gentle as well as effective, and for the most part safer in terms of side effects when used appropriately. Another benefit of botanical medicines is the comprehensiveness and complexity of each medicinal plant. Because of the many diverse constituents all working together, a single plant may have multiple healing properties simultaneously. In this way, plant medicines favor whole health rather than just alleviate isolated symptoms. Health-care providers trained in the use of botanical medicines often prescribe healing plants by matching the unique needs of the individual with the special attributes of each plant.

Most of the medical literature offers a scientific and evidence-based approach for prescribing botanical medicines to treat people for their illnesses. Research reveals much about chemical constituents and clinical trials using plants as medicines, often times to compare with or take the place of pharmaceutical medications. It is simpler to view plants in this uncluttered way. It is also easier to use plants as medicines from the perspective of single properties for single conditions. There is, of course, the alternative perspective of using plants in a more comprehensive and artistic way, based on experience with plant medicines and intuition with people's needs. This model offers a more creative and holistic approach to treating people based on what makes each person unique. It allows practitioners to treat the individual, not the disease. This sort of practice necessitates a skillful practitioner to create custom herbal formulas and to guide the patient on how to use the prescribed medicinal plants.

The plants reviewed in the scope of this text are relatively safe for most to take at home. But any medicine, including "natural medicine," is best taken under the supervision and guidance of an expert in the field. This ensures higher efficacy and better safety, especially for women who are pregnant or lactating.

While the number of botanical medicines used to treat those afflicted with fatigue is too enormous to capture, it is important to look at those in particular which have been well-studied for their role in reducing chronic fatigue. The herbal medicines that have been evaluated for this use tend to fall into one of four categories: antioxidants that reduce oxidative damage found in CFS, immunomodulating plants that support and normalize the immune dysfunction, adaptogenic herbs that modulate the adrenal-stress response, and the mood-uplifting herbs that help improve mental and emotional well-being.

BOTANICAL ANTIOXIDANTS

Research has repeatedly suggested that oxidative stress contributes to the pathology and clinical symptoms of CFS. Oxidative stress is damage created by the generation of free radicals, also known as reactive oxygen species, that disrupt cellular structures. In CFS, mitochondrial dysfunction generates higher than normal amounts of free radicals. When mitochondria fail to work effectively, the cells cannot produce the energy needed to sustain life. The oxidative damage induced by improper mitochondrial activity leads to symptoms of fatigue, muscle pain, malaise, postexercise lethargy, and even immune system dysfunction, all characteristics of CFS. Also in CFS, enzymes needed to reduce the effects of oxidative damage tend to be in short supply, further exacerbating this vicious cycle. One way to reverse this process is to support the body with high doses of antioxidants. Plants and plant foods provide most of the exogenous antioxidants needed to control free radical damage, and medicinal botanicals can also increase the body's production and activity of enzymes that control oxidative stress. The plants described in this text are relatively safe—they have been used for centuries and they have research to support their profound antioxidant capabilities. Some can be included into the diet, others taken in medicinal doses as prescribed accordingly.

Hypericum (Saint John's Wort)

While native to Europe, this little plant can be found growing almost like a weed in meadows and along the side of roads in North America. It is named after John the Baptist, since it tends to bloom toward the end of June, around the time of his birthday. Conventionally thought of as an herbal antidepressant, St John's wort has so many medicinal qualities in addition to mood support. This plant has been proposed in several studies for its use in treating those with CFS.[1,2] Mice induced with chronic fatigue experienced decreased levels of glutathione reductase and superoxide dismutase, two enzymes needed for controlling oxidative damage. Administration of St John's wort normalized these enzymes while stabilizing the effects of oxidative damage. Typically for use in mood elevation, St John's wort is used in dosages of 300 mg three times daily. It will be interesting to see actual human clinical trials using this herb for CFS, and at what dosages it will be most effective.

St John's wort dosages:

• Standardized extract in capsule form: 300 mg three times daily for at least 3 to 4 weeks

Vaccinium myrtillus (Bilberry and Blueberry)

Bilberry has been used for centuries, both medicinally and as a food in jams and pies. It is related to the blueberry and is native to Northern Europe. Historically, bilberries have been eaten in the forms of extracts, pies, and jams by people with retinopathies and difficulty with vision. Not long ago, bilberry jam was very popular during World War II for pilots in the British Royal Air Force, improving visual acuity as well as night vision.

The fruits and leaves of this plant contain many nutrient-rich substances, which also have biochemical effects in the body. One of the most common of these substances, a group of pigmented molecules called anthocyanidins, give bilberries their blue-violet color. Anthocyanidins exert multiple physiological effects in the body. They help increase the production of glycosaminoglycans, proteins necessary for building and maintaining joints and cartilage. They can decrease permeability of blood vessels, reducing the tendency for edema and tissue fluid accumulation. And they also calm down inflammatory processes, making them useful for treating people with ulcers and gastric disorders by protecting the lining of the digestive tract.[3] Bilberry also contains many other chemicals and minerals that traditionally and currently are used for cardiovascular disease, circulatory disorders, diabetes, and high cholesterol.[4] These include the flavonoids, tannins, polyphenols, and even chromium.[5,6]

Blueberries, a cousin of the bilberry, provide additional nourishment. Blueberry fruit is high in fiber and antioxidants such as vitamin C, beta-carotene, glutathione, and alpha-tocopherol (vitamin E). It also contains anti-inflammatory compounds such as ellagitannins, flavonols, quercetin, catechins, and phenolic acids.[7] There are over twenty-five individual anthocyanidins in blueberry fruit.[8,9,10]

These very chemicals make bilberries and blueberries powerful sources of antioxidants as well. In fact, it is commonly known now that a diet rich in fruits and vegetables provides much of the antioxidants needed to slow down the aging process and reduce oxidative damage, which contributes to so many chronic illnesses. High fruit and vegetable intake can indeed increase antioxidant capacity which can be measured using an oxygen radical absorbance capacity (ORAC) assay.[11] Out of thirty fruits and vegetables tested in one study, the Vaccinium species (Bilberry and Blueberry) were found to have the highest ORAC scores.[12,13] They also had the highest combined anthocyanidin, phenol, and ORAC scores combined together.[14]

In treating those with CFS, bilberries may be of great benefit due to their high antioxidant potential[14] and specifically for their ability to enhance red blood cell resistance against oxidative damage.[15] While no studies to date have evaluated the use of Vaccinium in treatment of people with CFS, there is definite indication that this fruit's benefits are warranted. In a double-blind crossover study of people suffering from fibromyalgia, a related condition to CFS, individuals taking 80 mg of anthocyanidins daily had a small but clinically significant advantage over the placebo group.[16] They reported improved sleep and less fatigue, symptoms common to both fibromyalgia and CFS. It would be very confirming to see a similar study on those with CFS to show antioxidant benefits from anthocyanidins. However, given the high level of safety of this fruit, and the positive effects of its chemical constituents, a diet high in bilberries and blueberries would be the very minimum recommendation.

Supplementation, using extracts, teas, dried berries, powdered leaves, and berries in capsule form, would also be highly advisable. A typical dose of the dried, ripe berries is 20 to 60 mg daily (up to 320 mg) of the standardized bilberry extract with 25 percent anthocyanidin content.[17] Conversely, a tea may be prepared by adding 5 to 10 grams, 1 to 2 teaspoons, of mashed berries in cold water, bringing the water to a simmer for 10 minutes, and then straining. Clinical studies of Vaccinium species' effectiveness have used formulations containing 25 percent of the bioflavonoid complex anthocyanoside. Bilberry fruit and extract are considered generally safe, with no known side effects. However, bilberry leaf and extract should not be taken in large quantities over an extended period of time because the tannins they contain may become toxic.

Bilberry and Blueberry dosages:

- 20 to 60 mg (up to 320 mg) with 25 percent anthocyanidin content daily
- 5 to 10 grams or 1 to 2 tsp of mashed or dried berries per cup of boiling water

Sambucus nigra (Elderberry)

Elderberries are another darkly pigmented fruit with similar medicinal properties as the Vaccinium species of blueberries and bilberries. Anthocyanins are among the most abundant flavonoids found in elderberries but that is not to overshadow other constituents such as rutin, tannins, essential oils, and hyperosides which support the immune system, reduce inflammation, and control the allergic response.[18,19,20,21,22,23] Because elderberry increases production of inflammatory cytokines like interleukins and tumor necrosis factor, it is known to be an immune enhancing botanical as well.[24] In fact, it has been used historically to cure infections caused by viruses, including colds, influenza, and fevers. It also has antibacterial and antifungal properties making it useful for treating boils, wounds, and other types of skin inflammatory conditions. Elderberry especially seeks out to destroy viruses, and has been found very effective against several strains of the flu virus.[25] This herb can be used for those with CFS who have viral origins, as well as generalized immune dysregulation. It can also be a potent antioxidant source for reducing oxidative stress.

For treatment of influenza, 15 mL up to four times daily of elderberry juice extract has been used, with about half that frequency in children.[25] A similar protocol can be used for treating individuals with CFS. Only commercially prepared extracts of elderberry should be taken—the raw berries and bark of the tree are toxic and should not be consumed!

Elderberry dosages:

- 15 mL elderberry juice or extract up to four times daily during acute infections

Vitis vinifera (Grape)

Grapes have been heralded for thousands of years in Greek, Egyptian, and other Mediterranean cultures where they grow natively. They were enjoyed both as delicious fruits, sumptuous wines, and of course medicinal plants. The healing values of grapes have been honored by Greek philosophers in the form of wine, but many Europeans also used other parts of the grape besides the fruit. Some made ointments from grapevine sap for treating skin diseases and disorders of the eyes. The leaves were used to stop hemorrhaging, and reduce inflammation leading to pain, making this plant a popular remedy for hemorrhoids. Raisins, dried grapes, are still commonly used for relieving constipation, while the ripe whole fruits were traditionally also used for cancer, cholera, smallpox, nausea, eye infections, and skin, kidney, and liver diseases.[26,27]

While the whole fruit contains many healing properties, research is now showing that many of these medicinal qualities come from the seeds themselves. They contain vitamin E, flavonoids, linoleic acid, and most famously, compounds called procyanidins including tannins, pycnogenols, and oligomeric proanthocyanidins (OPCs).[28] These active constituents can also be found in lower concentrations in the skin of the grape, which contains higher amounts of resveratrol, a popular antiaging medicine. Procyanidins, pycnogenols, OPCs, and resveratrol contribute most of the antioxidant benefits of grapes.[28] So it is very important when increasing grape intake in the diet to consume those with their skins and seeds intact (and avoid seedless varieties).

Like blueberries and bilberries, grapes get their dark purple color from chemicals called anthocyanidins and proanthocyanidins (precursors to the former).[29] In addition, the fruit, fruit skin, seeds, and leaves of grapes hold medicinal properties. They provide flavonoids, quercetin, catechin, myricetin, and kaemferol. These compounds can reduce platelet aggregation in arterial plaques, cause dilation of atherosclerotic blood vessels, and lower the oxidation of LDL cholesterol, the low-density lipoprotein responsible for increasing risk of heart disease.[30,31,32] All of these actions validate the tradition of drinking a glass of wine to reduce heart disease. In fact, proanthocyanidins from grape seeds can decrease reperfusion injury after heart muscle tissue is deprived of oxygen during a heart attack.[33] But it is not just red wine that benefits the heart. Any intake of myricetin, kaemferol, and quercetin from grape seeds and fruit can reduce the risk of coronary heart disease.[34]

The phenolic compounds such as OPCs grant grapes their high antioxidant capabilities.[31] Not surprisingly, the higher the proanthocyanidin content, the better the antioxidant activity of grape products.[29] The OPCs and flavonoids enhance antioxidant activity in the body partially by lowering levels of superoxide, a type of free radical. Studies using extracts of 300 mg of grape seed proanthocyanidins show increased antioxidant activity in healthy people.[32] Another study found that OPCs from grape seeds are better at protecting against oxidative stress and free radical damage than combinations of vitamins E, C, and beta-carotene.[35] Grape OPCs can prevent against oxidation of lipids and consequent damage to DNA, as this has been shown to be a problem for those with CFS. These types of benefits can prevent and treat oxidative stress in individuals with CFS.

An effective dose would be 360 to 720 mg daily of grape seed extracts. For protection against oxidative stress, make sure that the standardized extract contains 40 to 80 percent proanthocyanidins or 95 percent OPC value. As mentioned earlier, the high safety of this fruit makes it an easy recommendation to most and a welcome addition into a healthful diet already rich in fruits and vegetables. It is important to note the benefits of the seeds themselves and to eat grapes that still contain the seeds in their natural form instead of those altered to grow without their seeds.

Grape dosages:

- 360 to 720 mg of grape seed extract containing 40 to 80 percent proanthocyanidins or 95 percent OPC.

Camellia sinensis (Green Tea)

Perhaps one of the oldest time-honored traditions is the ritual of drinking tea. In India and China, this tradition goes back thousands of years ago, when people first thought to steep tea leaves in boiling water to bring out their medicinal qualities. A popular beverage even today, green tea is consumed by people all over the world. It was originally used as a mental stimulant, a diuretic used to promote urine excretion, and as an astringent to control bleeding. It is still used for those reasons today, among other ones such as reducing gas and bloating, improving digestion, and regulating body temperature and blood sugar. Green tea is made from unfermented leaves and contains powerful antioxidants called polyphenols which are among its most important medicinal properties.

Green tea has been gaining popularity more recently for its many medicinal properties. Its ability to protect the cartilage in joints by inhibiting breakdown of proteoglycans and collagen gives it some credibility for usage in the treatment of arthritis.[36,37] Another well-studied use of green tea is in preventing and treating cancers. The polyphenols protect DNA against damage, stimulate tumor cell death, and support overall antimutagenic processes.[38,39,40,41,42,43] Also, green tea prevents skin inflammation and UV radiation-induced damage leading to skin cancers.[44] Due to its small but significant caffeine content, which accelerates resting energy expenditures, green tea may be useful in weight loss.[45,46,47] Its extract increases metabolism of fats and calories in general, while curbing appetite. Additionally, this medicinal beverage is found to protect against Alzheimer's disease,[48] prevent loss of bone mineral density associated with osteoporosis,[49] and reduce dental disease from bacterial overgrowth.[50]

These are just a few of the many impressive qualities of green tea. But perhaps one of its most effective uses is that as an antioxidant. All of the arial parts of the plant, the leaf bud, leaf, and stem, can be steamed at high temperatures to produce the highly polyphenolic green tea commonly enjoyed. These polyphenols include flavonoids, phenolic acids, epigallocatechin gallate (EGCG) and other catechins, all of which are said to offer many benefits.[51,52,53] Flavonoids and EGCG are powerful antioxidants which reduce oxidation of lipids and cholesterols. They also prevent DNA damage by reducing free radical generation, serving as another means by which to lower oxidative stress.[54,55,56] Another added side benefit of green tea is that it can increase the body's concentrations of Lactobacillus and Bifidobacteria,[57] both of which can support the immune system, improve the balance of essential fatty acids, and reduce overall oxidation levels. All of these benefits are very much needed for individuals with CFS.

A study of mice induced with CFS showed the positive effects of using green tea extract containing catechins.[58] Mice forced to swim daily presented with elevated levels of lipid peroxidation and lowered levels of glutathione, signs of oxidative stress. Using green tea extract and catechin daily for 1 week brought lipid peroxidation back to normal and restored the dwindling glutathione levels. While it would not be appropriate to extrapolate dosages of green tea and catechins from this mouse-model, it seems very important to evaluate the use of green tea extract in the treatment of CFS.

For most, since this medicinal herb is very safe, green tea can be consumed in amounts of one to three cups daily as it is in many Asian cultures. In a standardized extract form, the recommended dose is 300 to 400 mg daily with 240 to 320 mg of polyphenol content. Children might find green tea to be too stimulating, so it should be used only in very small amounts if at all. Because of the small but potent caffeine content in green tea, people with anxiety, heart palpitations, kidney disease, and stomach ulcers should avoid green tea. Excessive caffeine intake over long periods of time can induce a state of overactivity and hyperalertness. Excessive amounts of green tea can deliver enough caffeine to induce irritability, insomnia, dizziness, and heart palpitations. Because of this, pregnant and breastfeeding woman should consume no more than one cup of green tea a day, or better yet avoid it altogether.

Green tea dosages:

- 1 to 2 tsp of dried green tea herb per cup of boiling water, drunk 3 to 4 times daily
- 300 to 400 mg standardized extract with 240 to 320 mg polyphenol content daily.

Emblica officinalis (Amla Fruit or Indian Gooseberry)

Amla fruit is one of the most famous of Ayurvedic herbs for its strength as a rejuvenating tonic. It imparts strength and resilience not only to those who are debilitated with illness but also for those who are in a healthy state. Amla is the most abundant ingredient in a popular Ayurvedic rejuvenative jam called "Chyawanprash." This jam is eaten daily by children, elderly people, and healthy individuals alike for reversing the aging process and strengthening the immune system. It is known to clear the eyes and improve vision, as well as treat premature gray hair. Traditionally, the fruits of this plant were used for a variety of inflammatory conditions such as gastritis, hemorrhoids, colitis, and musculoskeletal pain. This powerful antiinflammatory property has been confirmed in research as well.[59] In addition, there is evidence of Amla's ability to support learning and memory. Given to mice in one experiment, it was found to improve memory scores and reverse amnesia by acting on the neurotransmitter functions in the brain.[60]

The taste of this fruit is unforgettably sour due to its very high concentration of ascorbic acid (vitamin C). Interestingly, an Ayurvedic method of preparation has been found to improve the vitamin C content in Amla even further.[61] While increasing the ascorbic acid content, which accounts for 45 to 70 percent of the total antioxidant activity, this processing technique boosts Amla's ability to quench free radicals and reduce oxidative stress.

The amazing antioxidant and free-radical scavenging properties of this plant cannot be understated. It can significantly reduce lipid peroxidation in streptozotocin-induced diabetic rats with high levels of oxidative damage.[62] The plant phenolic compounds in extracts are equivalent to 33 to 44 percent gallic acid, the same substance that makes green tea such a strong source of antioxidants.[63] These, and other, compounds can restore the activities of enzymes that reduce the effects of oxidative damage in the brain: superoxide dismutase, catalase, and glutathione peroxidase. So the antistress benefits of Amla may be due to its ability to reduce the byproducts of oxidation occurring from stress.[64] Some of the compounds responsible for this restorative action are categorized as tannins.[65] There is also evidence that these tannins protect against the deterioration of vitamin C, allowing this vitamin's activities to last longer as well.[66] These antioxidant effects give credence to Amla's value in antiaging formulas[67] for its ability to reverse the effects of chronic disease.

Another benefit of Amla is its ability to moderate the immune system functions. While human studies have yet to be done on this subject, there is evidence that this fruit can increase output of certain immune cellular components. It seems to double the numbers of natural killer cells (NK cells), while also enhancing their activity to kill tumor cells (and potentially viruses and other microorganisms too).[68] It also enhances antibody-dependent cellular cytotoxicity, a process that destroys foreign microbes and abnormal body cells. These two factors helped improve lifespan by 35 percent longer in mice infected with tumor cells. Amla can be very beneficial in the treatment of CFS, especially among those who suffer from immune dysfunction characterized by low NK cell activity.

Amla dosage:

- 1 to 3 tsp of Chyawanprash jam daily.

IMMUNE-SUPPORTIVE HERBS

As discussed in an earlier chapter, one of the many proposed etiologies of CFS has to do with dysfunction of the immune system. The immune system may be suboptimal or deficient; research suggests that NK cell activity is reduced in CFS, rendering the body's defense against viruses and bacteria inadequate. On the other hand, many other immune cells are excessively active or exaggerated. For example, some people with CFS are found to have disproportionately higher levels of helper (T4) and cytotoxic (T8) lymphocytes. Elevated cytokines, chemical mediators of immune and inflammatory responses, are also common. Many of these immune abnormalities resemble those observed in people with chronic viral illnesses, and many researchers believe there to be correlations between CFS, immune dysfunction, and viral infections. Regardless of exactly how these associations work, CFS is starting to be known as a type of "polycellular immune dysfunction" due to the multiple immune cell abnormalities occurring concurrently.

As a condition affecting the immune system in various—often opposite or conflicting—ways, CFS becomes even more difficult to treat using medicines that induce only one type of immune cell function. In other words, it does not make sense to treat someone with CFS using only an antiviral medication protocol while ignoring the overall immune system dysfunction. Nor would it be wise to overly stimulate the immune system if its activity seems excessive or exaggerated to begin with. Instead, it is preferable to treat each individual with CFS using a unique comprehensive immune-modulating approach by supporting the weaker areas while calming down the overactive ones. While standard pharmaceutical medications are not designed to achieve this type of goal, botanical medicines can offer a more holistic approach aimed at normalizing and optimizing immune function.

Echinacea species (Purple Coneflower)

Named after its prickly spines that cover the seed head central in the flower, Echinacea comes from the Greek word "echinos" for hedgehog. Historically, this herb was considered a "cure-all" by Native Americans, used thereafter to treat scarlet fever, syphilis, malaria, diphtheria, and blood poisoning from infections. Much of the modern usage and research on Echinacea occurs in Germany, where this plant is very popular as an immune tonic.

Purple coneflower is a plant that could be one of three main species of Echinacea: E. angustifolia, E. pallida, and E. purpurea. The whole plant was used, including the roots as well as the aerial parts (flowers, leaves, and stems) for different purposes. These plants are native to North America and were used as traditional herbal remedies by the Great Plains Indian tribes before being adopted for medicinal use by settlers. For a long time, Echinacea species was used for treatment of wounds, sores, snakebites, spider bites, toothaches, burns, and even cancers.[26] In fact, E. angustifolia and E. pallida were officially written into the U.S. National Formulary for prescribed medical uses from 1916 to 1950 until the antibiotic revolution gained popularity over them.[69] Now, with increasing emergence of antibiotic resistance, Echinacea's use against microorganisms that cause infections has made a comeback. Its active components include, but are not limited to, flavonoids, polysaccharides, alkylamides, heteroxylan, and arabinogalactan.

Commonly used for treating and preventing respiratory tract infections due to colds and influenza, Echinacea serves as an important immune system modulator, rendering it very useful for correcting the immune dysfunction found in CFS. Clinically, Echinacea exerts many effects on the immune system. It stimulates a nonspecific immune response by promoting the release of tumor necrosis factor, interleukin-1, and interferon.[69,70,71] These factors help increase overall lymphocyte activity of T cells and B cells, as well as increasing phagocytosis, the ability to engulf pathogens and destroy microorganisms such as viruses and bacteria that cause disease. Additionally, Echinacea exerts an anti-inflammatory effect by inhibiting cyclooxygenase and 5-lipogenase.[72,73]

In a study using E. purpurea extract on healthy volunteers and individuals with CFS, the extract significantly enhanced the function and activity of NK cells in both groups.[74] This is impressive as the scientific literature indicates reduced NK cell activity and numbers in individuals with CFS. Echinacea also significantly increased the antibody-dependent cellular cytotoxicity against cells infected with HHV6 virus. It seems that one effect of Echinacea is to stimulate circulation of immune cells into the peripheral bloodstream to target pathogens. In this way, extract of E. purpurea enhanced the immune function in healthy individuals as well as those with depressed activity and CFS.

For immune-modulating purposes, dosages may vary considerably. Freeze-dried Echinacea extract can be given at 100 to 300 mg capsules containing 4 percent phenolics three times daily.[75] A liquid herb juice preparation of twenty drops every few hours during acute infection, followed by half that dose three times daily is useful for most viral illnesses.[76] The root can be preserved in tincture form using grain alcohol or glycerine, and administered in doses up to 2 to 3 mL three times daily for short periods of time.[77] The safest route of intake is to prepare a tea by steeping 1 to 2 grams of dried root or herb in 8 ounces of boiling water for 15 minutes, and then drinking one to four cups daily for long-term benefit.[78]

No matter the dosage, Echinacea tends to work best if given in 8-week increments, followed by a week of hiatus before restarting.[79] Children's herbal dosages are calculated by dividing the child's weight by 150 lb (70 kg) and using this fraction of the adult dosage. Echinacea is rated as a safe herb when used as instructed on the product label and under the guidance of a trained health professional. However, there are some issues to consider. Some individuals with atopic conditions may have allergic reactions to Echinacea, so it is best to consult with a clinician before use. Also, Echinacea is contraindicated in those with concomitant autoimmune conditions such as Graves' disease, Hashimoto's thyroiditis, and multiple sclerosis due to its immune stimulating properties. Individuals with possible autoimmune disease should also consult a clinician well versed in the field of botanical medicine before starting a treatment plan including Echinacea. This herb should not be used in people with tuberculosis, leukemia, diabetes, multiple sclerosis, HIV, and AIDS due to its potent immune stimulating effects. For this reason, organ transplant recipients taking immunosuppressive medications should also avoid this herb. This herb is relatively safe to use during pregnancy despite some claims about risks of birth defects, but again, pregnant women should consult their prenatal physicians before commencing treatment with Echinacea.

Echinacea dosages:

- Freeze-dried extract 100 to 300 mg capsules containing 4 percent phenolics three times daily
- Liquid herb juice twenty drops every hour during active infections
- 2 to 3 mL three times daily of the tincture (preserved in alcohol)
- 1 to 2 grams of dried root or herb in 8 ounces of boiling water drunk as a tea three times daily
- Always take a week-long break from Echinacea treatment every 8 weeks before resuming.

Astragalus membranaceous (Milkvetch and Huang-qi)

Astragalus is a hardy perennial herb whose root has been used for thousands of years in Chinese medicine as a spleen and blood tonic, to strengthen the body against disease. It grows in China, Korea, and Mongolia. The roots are harvested off plants that are at least 4 years old. As it also grows in North America, it has been used in traditional native medicine for coughs, fever, chest and back pain, high blood pressure, diabetes, and liver disease.[26]

The root contains flavonoids, saponins that bind to toxins for excretion, trace minerals, amino acids, and other constituents acting as antioxidants.[80,81] Currently, this herbal medicine is included in many immune supportive formulations for conditions such as respiratory infections, cancer, AIDS, and other forms of immune compromise. It seems to have an affinity for the immune system in that its active constituents activate B lymphocytes (to produce antibodies against pathogens) and macrophages to engulf those foreign microbes.[82] It can also enhance the effects of many other immune factors, while improving the response of T lymphocytes which might be suppressed in conditions with abnormal immune function.[83,84] Astragalus also has antibacterial, antiviral, and anti-inflammatory effects as well.

While there are no studies on using Astragalus for treatment of those with CFS, it seems that its immune modulating effects in studies of people with AIDS can be relatable or applicable to those with other conditions with viral origins. When used appropriately, it may help to reduce severity of virally induced conditions such as CFS, especially in individuals with multiple immune abnormalities.

General immune enhancing effects can occur with dosages of 4 to 7 grams Astragalus root daily for short periods of time.[85,86] No more than 28 grams daily should be used, as some research suggests that this higher dose may counteract the benefits by inducing immune suppression.[86] This medicinal herb is commonly enjoyed in Asian cuisine mixed into soups with other ingredients such as mushrooms and other herbs for immune support. The following are other methods of administration.

Astragalus dosages:

- Decoction (strong boiled tea): 3 to 6 grams of dried root boiled for 15 minutes in 12 ounces of water, three times per day
- Fluid extract (1:1) in 25 percent ethanol: 2 to 4 mL three times a day
- Powdered root: 500 to 1,000 mg three or four times per day
- Powdered extract (solid): 100 to 150 mg of a product standardized to 0.5 percent 4-hydroxy-3-methoxy isoflavone. *Note:* this chemical is used only as a manufacturing marker, not as a guarantee of potency or effectiveness
- Tincture (1:5) in 30 percent ethanol: 3 to 5 mL three times a day.

Ganoderma lucidum and Lentinus edodes
(Reishi and Shiitake Mushrooms)

Reishi and Shiitake mushrooms have been revered as potent medicines in China and Japan for thousands of years. Their long history of use in traditional medicine prompted modern research studies to explore their immune enhancing qualities. Currently, extracts of these mushrooms are used all over Asia as anti-cancer therapies, approved by the national governments for clinical use. Their popularity is rising in the United States as well. They can be enjoyed as part of the Asian cuisine, eaten cooked in soups and stir-frys, however their best medic-inal properties require higher dosages in extract forms or injectables for ideal absorption.

Active constituents of medicinal mushrooms such as Reishi and Shiitake in-clude polysaccharides, long chains of sugar molecules that activate macrophages and lymphocytes. These compounds have medicinal properties as antioxidants, antitumor, antiviral, and immune modulating effects.[87] In fact, they stimulate functioning of macrophages and T lymphocytes by increasing their production and release of cytokines.[88] They also significantly increase NK cell activity.[89] For these reasons, Reishi extracts are given as treatment for people with advanced cancer in Japan. To top that, the peptides, or protein molecules, found in Reishi mushrooms also offer potent antioxidant qualities.[90] The ability to fight off viruses, improve NK cell activity, and stimulate better functioning of T lymphocytes and macrophages makes this mushroom an ideal plant medicine for use in the treat-ment of CFS. Reishi is typically dosed at 1.5 grams daily up to 9 grams total of the crude dried mushroom, or 1.5 grams daily of Reishi powder. It can also be absorbed in liquid form, preserved in alcohol, dosed at 1 mL daily of the Reishi tincture.

Shiitake mushrooms also contain a certain type of immune supportive polysac-charide called lentinans. In one study, lentinans extracted from shiitake mush-rooms dramatically increased NK cells and their activity in individuals with CFS. Those given the extract showed a tripling of their NK cells along with significant improvements in their sense of well-being and energy levels![91] Another study showed improved NK cell activity and antibody-dependent cellular cytotoxicity in patients with fatigue due to low NK cell syndrome.[92] Now since lentinan does not get absorbed thoroughly with oral intake, it needs to first be prepared in extract form to be administered by injection. The researchers in the previously mentioned studies used injections of 1 mg every other day to achieve their pos-itive results. Another way of administering this mushroom therapeutically is to extract it using alcohol. This formulation, called peptidomannan or KS-2, binds the polysaccharide to amino acids, making it more absorbable. It is dosed at 75 to 150 mg three times daily for up to 8 weeks at a time. This makes it ideal for use during acute infectious illnesses and flare-ups of CFS immune symptoms.[92]

Reishi dosages:

- $1\frac{1}{2}$ grams up to 9 grams daily of crude dried herb
- $1\frac{1}{2}$ grams dried herb powder daily

- 1 mL of alcohol-preserved tincture daily

Shiitake dosages:

- 75 to 150 mg of alcohol preserved tincture three times daily for up to 8 weeks at a time.

Uncaria tomentosa (Cat's Claw or Una de Gato)

Cat's claw is named for it hook-like thorns on its vines. It is native to the Amazon rainforests as well as tropical forests in Central and South America. Traditionally, it has been used since the era of the Incas for healing arthritis, reducing inflammation and fever, and soothing stomach ulcers and dysentery.[93]

Cat's claw has been gaining interest more recently for its overall anti-inflammatory effects. This plant's medicinal properties lie in the root and bark and its major active constituent is an alkaloid chemical called rhynchophylline. This and other pentacyclic oxindole alkaloids found in Cat's claw confer its immunomodulating effects by enhancing macrophage activity and lymphocyte activity.[94,95] This medicinal plant seems to prolong the survival time for white blood cells such as NK cells, B and T lymphocytes, and granulocytes.[96] It also has potent antioxidant and antiviral effects,[97,98] making it dually purposeful for treating those with CFS. Because of the antagonistic effects of another chemical compound found in Cat's claw, the tetracyclic oxindole alkaloids (TOAs), it is important to choose only TOA-free Cat's claw extract.

Cat's claw seems to have relatively few side effects, namely dizziness, nausea, and diarrhea, which tend to self-resolve with continued use of the herb. Typical doses for immune support range from 20 to 150 mg three times daily of dry standardized extract.[94] A tincture of the herb preserved in alcohol and water can be taken in dosages of $^1/_4$ to $^1/_2$ teaspoonfuls three times daily. Or the root bark can be brewed as a tea using 1 to 10 grams of the dry herb boiled for 15 minutes in 8 ounces of water. The tea should be strained, cooled, and drunk up to three times daily. Avoid giving Cat's claw to children until further research is done to evaluate the effects in youngsters.

Cat's claw dosages:

- 20 to 150 mg dry standardized extract up to three times daily
- $^1/_4$ to $^1/_2$ tsp of alcoholic tincture of herb up to three times daily
- 1 to 10 grams of dry herb boiled in 8 ounces of water, up to three cups of tea daily.

Panax Ginseng (Panax, Korean, Chinese ginseng)

P. ginseng is a family of plants whose roots are legendary over thousands of years for their ability to support stress resistance. While most of the beneficial qualities of Panax are described in the Adaptogenic Botanicals section, it is important not to overlook its powerful immune supporting functions. In fact, Panax has been known to increase NK cell activity, macrophage function, and interferon production, working across many different levels of the immune system. It enables macrophages to help other lymphocytes to locate and destroy viruses, bacteria, and even cancer cells.[99]

In a clinical study of twenty healthy volunteers, one group was treated with 100 mg of Panax aqueous extract twice daily for 8 weeks, while another group was given the same amount in standardized extract, and the rest were given placebo.[100] After treatment, blood samples were checked for various immune parameters. Those treated with Panax demonstrated improvements in their numbers of helper T-lymphocytes, subsets of T4/T8, NK cell activity, and total lymphocyte output. They also had benefits on the functions of these immune cells. They had increased ability of a type of white blood cell (neutrophil) to gravitate toward pathogens and engulf and destroy them. These beneficial effects started just after 4 weeks of treatment and continued even at 8 weeks.

American ginseng (*P. quinquefolium*) is a slightly different variety of Panax. While it may have similar stress resistant characteristics, it is better known for its immune supportive actions. The polysaccharides (complex sugar molecules) appear to confer its immunomodulating effects.[101] American ginseng stimulates monocytes, tumor necrosis factor (TNF)-alpha, interferon-gamma, as well as NK cell activity, interleukin-2 (IL-2), and other factors involved in cell-mediated immunity.[101,102,103] It also seems to stimulate B-lymphocyte proliferation, serum immunoglobulin production, and macrophage production of IL-1 and IL-6.[104] Panax, like several other botanicals, plays an important role in promoting the immune system and should be considered in the treatment of those with CFS of viral or immune dysfunction origins.

The usual dose of Panax is 15 mg of standardized ginsenosides or saponins in extract form, administered up to three times daily. Like Siberian ginseng, it is important to take intervals in long-term use. Panax can be taken daily for 2 to 3 weeks, with a 2-week rest period before resuming treatment. Excessive dosages can cause similar symptoms to that of Siberian ginseng—insomnia, anxiety, and others such as breast pain and menstrual irregularities.

P. ginseng dosages:

• 15 mg standardized ginsenosides up to three times daily for 3 weeks on, 2 weeks off, 3 weeks on again.

ADAPTOGENIC BOTANICALS

Human beings are constantly being bombarded with stressful experiences. Whether these stresses are related to physical overwork, or mental fatigue, or emotional distress, the body reacts to all of them in the same familiar patterned response. Dr. Hans Selye explained this response to stress as a general adaptation syndrome in the 1930s.[105] His theory allowed us to view the stress response in light of the complex hormonal and neural pathways involved to help the body compensate. Some of the adrenal, pituitary, and hypothalamic hormonal responses to stress have already been reviewed in terms of their connections to CFS. For people with CFS, the stress response may be altered or exaggerated. They might have a blunted release of pituitary hormone ACTH, causing inadequate amounts of cortisol production by the adrenal glands. There may also be issues regarding the body's output of aldosterone and vasopressin, hormones involved in maintaining blood pressure and fluid balance during acute stressful onslaughts. One way to normalize the altered stress response is through the use of adaptogenic botanical medicines for nourishing the body during times of stress.

The term "adaptogen" was coined a few decades ago by a couple of doctors, Israel I. Brekhman and I.V. Dardymov, to describe substances with the ability to help the body resist or overcome stressors on the physical, chemical, emotional, and environmental levels.[106] For a plant to be called an adaptogen, it needed to be "innocuous" and have a "nonspecific, normalizing action." The modern understanding is that any safe plant that gives the body more resolve, allowing the body to better cope with stress, is an adaptogen. Most botanical adaptogens are considered "tonics" to the adrenal glands. The effects of botanical adaptogens often then trickle out through the connections among other neuroendocrine glands all throughout the body, especially those in the brain—the hypothalamus and pituitary. Herbal medicines that act as adaptogens strengthen the body to achieve better states of resistance to fatigue and burnout. They improve our ability to deal with stress and overcome challenges from a variety of life's situations. It is the nourishing effect combined with the invigorating effect that makes adaptogens so ideal for treating those with CFS.

Eleuthrococcus senticosis (Siberian Ginseng)

Siberian ginseng, called Eleuthro for short, is an ancient plant medicine used in China, Russia, Mongolia, and obviously, Siberia, where it is native. It has been greatly respected for its ability to restore vigor, improve memory, stimulate digestion, and promote a long life. In Russia, it has been extensively studied for its ability to help the body overcome stresses from the environment such as heat, cold, viruses and bacteria, pollution, and strain from overwork in extreme conditions. In China, it is used to promote the building of vital energy in the form of "qi" while controlling spleen and kidney deficiency conditions.

Siberian ginseng is probably one the most studied of all of the adaptogenic herbs. Many of the earlier studies of Siberian ginseng were conducted in Russia for evaluating athletic performance and endurance. Now, this herbal medicine is being researched for all kinds of conditions related to stress, fatigue, and chronic illness all over the world. The root of this plant has been revered for thousands of years in several traditional cultures of medicine for its overall rejuvenating and invigorating actions. The root contains phytochemicals, plant-based compounds that can act on various areas of the body. Most of these active compounds are grouped together as eleuthrosides. In addition, ginseng also contains chemicals such as saponins and lignans (to bind up toxic chemicals in the body), coumarins (to support healthy blood flow), and even nutrients such as vitamin E and beta-carotene.[107] Several of these constituents may be potent antioxidants, useful for preventing and treating cancer.[108] Siberian ginseng root has been found to increase lymphocyte counts and phagocyte activity,[109] rendering it a good immune-modulating herb as well. In some studies, Siberian ginseng daily for 1 month significantly increased helper T-cells and NK cell activity.[110] Studies have shown that this plant can reduce inflammation that causes chronic pain, while also inhibiting the activity of certain common viruses. These immune effects serve CFS sufferers well.

Ginseng's adaptogenic effects lie primarily in its influence over the pituitary-adrenocortical system.[111] It seems to support the body's ability to maintain normal cortisol levels in the blood by slowing down its metabolism in the liver. In CFS, it makes sense to extend the life of cortisol for those individuals unable to produce sufficient quantities. The longer the duration of cortisol's functions on the body, the less the burden on the adrenal glands to produce more. Lifting the workload off the adrenal glands may also reduce one aspect of the adrenal fatigue or burnout experienced.

Large clinical trials confirm this effect. A group of 2,100 healthy but stressed individuals were treated with Siberian ginseng root extract.[112] In this study, Siberian ginseng elicited several major benefits. It improved the subjects' ability to withstand adverse physical conditions such as heat, noise, motion, exercise, and workload increase. It also benefited the quality of exertion and athletic performance under stressful conditions. On the mental-emotional side, this herbal medicine boosted mental alertness, work output, and energy levels in the volunteers.

Not only did Siberian ginseng support healthy individuals, but it also showed adaptogenic effects on those with various disease states. The previously mentioned study also supported ginseng's effectiveness with improved resistance to physical hardships, increased performance under stressful environments, and better mental efficiency with higher energy. This arm of the study included over 2,200 individuals with cardiovascular conditions such as angina, hypertension, hypotension, rheumatic heart disease, as well as other disease states such as cancer, bronchitis, kidney disease, cerebral trauma, and several kinds of neuroses.

Siberian ginseng comes in a variety of different commercial forms, such as tincture, fluid extract, solid extract, and dried herb root. Typically, it is taken 1 to 3 times daily for up to 2 months at a time, after which it is generally a good idea to rest for 2 to 3 weeks before starting up the next long course. Ginseng is well-tolerated in most individuals at these dosages. Side effects may occur at dosages greater than six times the recommended amounts shown below. At these huge dosages, some may experience melancholy, anxiety, irritability, and insomnia.[112] Also, those with cardiovascular disease, such as rheumatic heart disease, may experience chest pain, palpitations, and elevated blood pressures at these significantly higher doses.

Siberian ginseng dosages:

- Dried root: 2 to 4 grams in tea or capsules daily
- Tincture (1:5): $\frac{1}{2}$ to 1 tsp three times daily
- Fluid extract (1:1): 2 to 4 mL

- Solid extract of dry, powdered root (20:1 or standardized to contain greater than 1 percent eleuthroside E): 100 to 200 mg twice daily
- All dosages should be taken 3 weeks on, 2 weeks off, then 3 weeks on again!

Panax species (Panax, Korean, Chinese, and American Ginsengs)

The Panax family has not been studied as extensively as the Siberian version of ginseng but its use is just as ancient and wrapped in many traditional cultures of medicines. Many believe it to be one of the most popular and famous medicinal plants in China and Korea. Again, the active compounds are found mainly in the root—the ginsenosides which have a wide range of pharmacological activity and effects. Unlike Siberian ginseng, only Panax family plants contain this particular group of chemicals, conferring an important difference between the two categories of ginsengs. This species of ginseng also contains pectin, B vitamins, and various flavonoids.[85] Together, these active constituents reduce platelet aggregation, stimulate nerve growth factors for neuroregeneration and protection of nerve tissues, and relax smooth muscles to open up bronchial airways in individuals with asthma.[113,114,115]

Just like Siberian ginseng, *P. ginseng* appears to stimulate NK cell activity and possibly other immune-system activity.[116] As a source of antioxidants, Panax is also known for its free radical scavenging effect to lower oxidative damage.[117,118]

As a potent adaptogen, the saponins found in *P. ginseng* appear to increase serum cortisol concentrations.[119,120] *P. ginseng* might also increase dehydroepiandrosterone sulfate (DHEA-S) levels in women.[121] Longevity of both DHEA-S and cortisol promote adrenal rest, improving resistance to stress. And the legends of its use as a tonic and rejuvenative are confirmed when using pure, high-quality extracts with known standardization of its active constituents.[122] In human clinical trials, Panax has shown dramatic improvements in those who are especially debilitated or feeble.[123] Treatment with Panax increases energy, mental and physical performance, while reducing the negative long-term effects of stress and consequences of high levels of stress hormones in the body. It also enhances liver function and protects against environmental toxic exposures such as radiation.

A great example of Panax's benefits on stress resistance can be seen in a study of male and female nurses switching their day-time work to night-time duties.[124] First, the nurses reported their own sense of well-being, mood, and competence. Next, they also underwent physical examinations and tests for mental performance, as well as laboratory tests for blood counts and blood chemistry. On various different measures, the nurses who were given Panax outperformed themselves and those given placebo. They showed improved mental and physical performance and overall energy.

Panax products range in quality, availability, and price. Unfortunately, many commercial products sold in the United States use low-grade sources such as smaller roots combined with other unusable chemicals, so they may not contain active ginsenosides. The best quality Panax products are prepared from old, wild, well-formed roots growing on good soil found in nature. These roots need to be at least 4 years old and the extracts should contain ideal ratios of ginsenosides (2:1 of Rb1:Rg1). Usual dose is 15 mg of standardized ginsenosides or saponins in extract form, administered up to three times daily. Like Siberian ginseng, it is important to take intervals in long-term use. Panax can be taken daily for 2 to 3 weeks, with a 2-week rest period before resuming treatment. Excessive dosages can cause similar symptoms to that of Siberian ginseng—insomnia, anxiety, and others such as breast pain and menstrual irregularities.

Panax ginseng dosages:

- 15 mg standardized ginsenosides up to three times daily for 3 weeks on, 2 weeks off, 3 weeks on again.

Rhodiola rosea (Rhodiola)

Rhodiola is commonly called roseroot or goldenroot and grows in harsh climates of Eastern Europe, Scandinavia, Siberia, Asia, and Alaska. It has been used medicinally since around the first century A.D. throughout these areas as a medicinal rejuvenating plant for its stimulating, anti-fatiguing and stress-resistant properties.[125] Its active constituents can be grouped mostly under a category of glycosides called salidroside, or also rhodioloside or rhodosine.[126] While this herb helps to activate the adrenal response to stress, it does not cause rebound fatigue. In fact, one study finds that Rhodiola "typically generates no side effects, unlike traditional stimulants that possess addiction, tolerance and abuse potential, produce a negative effect on sleep structure, and cause rebound hypersomnolence or 'come down' effects."[127] In clinical trials, it increases mental performance and physical working capacity, with effects starting within 30 minutes of administration and lasting for at least 4 to 6 hours. And contrary to most stimulating medicines that pump energy but rob sleep, Rhodiola actually seems to affect sleep in a positive way. In a study of twenty-four young men living at high altitudes for over 1 year, this herbal medicine matched acetazolamide in inducing restful sleep without the side effects of lethargy.[128]

Like many medicinal plants, Rhodiola also contains flavonoids and other antioxidant compounds. It can reduce lipid peroxidation by increasing the synthesis of glutathione in rats[129] as well as in humans[130] protecting cells and mitochondria from free radical damage. In animals, this plant offers protection from stressors such as cold, radiation, and increased workload. It also decreases work-induced fatigue and improves learning and memory.[125] Recently, a study on mice found that Rhodiola also works as an antidepressant and a calming botanical for anxiety.[131]

In addition, roseroot has been used extensively for building stamina in athletes, with numerous clinical studies originating in Eastern Europe and Russia since the 1960s. It is known to lengthen the time it takes to reach exhaustion from endurance training exercises by improving depth of breathing—balancing oxygen consumption and carbon dioxide release.[132] Research suggests that this improvement in stamina occurs on a cellular level. A rat study showed increased productivity of ATP, a biochemical fuel source, by the mitochondria, even in response to exhaustive exercise.[133] As an antiinflammatory herb, it can lower levels of C-reactive protein, a marker for inflammation. This protein level was lower in a group of healthy volunteers using Rhodiola for several days before and after exhausting exercise, compared to people who took placebo.[132]

Beyond its stamina-strengthening benefits, Rhodiola reduces fatigue and boosts cognitive performance. A group of researchers found interesting results in a double-blind crossover study of fifty-six young overworked physicians doing night duty.[125] Just 2 weeks of low-dose daily therapy with this botanical showed overall benefits in mental acuity involving complex perceptive and cognitive cerebral functions. Significant improvements were measured on five different tests of associative thinking, short-term memory, calculation and ability of concentration, and speed of audio-visual perception. No side effects were experienced by the subjects. This improvement in mental functioning may affect the ability to learn. Another study found that Rhodiola curbs fatigue and enhances mental work capacity in military cadets with constant underlying job strain.[134] Those cadets who took the herb regularly showed significantly less fatigue than the placebo group and this effect was statistically significant. Even in a rat experiment, Rhodiola extract in a single dose of 0.10 mL per rat improved learning and retention after 24 hours in a maze-method used for testing learning and adaptability. A 10-day treatment course of the same dosage also supports long-term memory.[135]

Another double-blind, randomized, and placebo-controlled study offered low dose Rhodiola extract for 20 days to foreign students during a stressful examination period.[136] Those taking the medicines showed significant benefit in physical fitness, mental fatigue, and neuromotor tests. These individuals also reported improved sense of well-being. The authors did not find significant improvements in their test scores, but they attributed that lack of positive change to the suboptimal dosages used.

As Rhodiola improves learning ability, cognitive functioning, and long-term memory, it may be one of the best botanical prescriptions for affecting mental decline in CFS. Its properties as an antioxidant, an antiinflammatory, and a stamina-builder by increasing ATP production in mitochondria during times of stress make it ideal for this condition as well. Most people can take Rhodiola without risking adverse effects, at dosages of 50 to 100 mg twice daily of either whole herb capsules or aqueous extract up to 4 weeks at a time, with a break of 1 week before starting the next course.

Rhodiola dosages:

- 50 to 100 mg of standardized herb capsules or aqueous extract (with 3 percent rosavins and 1 percent salidrosides) twice daily for 4 weeks, then 1 week rest before resuming treatment

Glycyrrhiza glabra (Licorice Root)

Licorice root has been used for thousands of years as a flavorful spice for its sweetness. This plant grows wild in Asia, parts of Europe, and also in the Americas. Medicinally, the root has been prized as a soothing demulcent (a coating agent) as well as a stimulating expectorant (an agent that rids mucus from the respiratory tract). In modern times, it is commonly used to relieve respiratory ailments (like sore throats, bronchitis, and asthma), stomach problems (like heartburn from acid reflux and ulcers), inflammatory disorders with pain and muscle spasms, skin diseases, stress burnout, and liver problems. It is also a strong antiviral medicine, making it useful for treatment of viral infections such as the flu, colds, hepatitis, urinary tract infections, and others.[26] Among these many medicinal uses, licorice root also has hormone balancing properties. Its ability to lower excessively elevated estrogen levels while improving progesterone levels makes it effective for treating conditions such as premenstrual syndrome (PMS).[137] Licorice might also have an effect on mental function and can lower anxiety. In a study of mice, aqueous extract of licorice significantly improved learning and memory.[138] It even counteracted the side effect of amnesia (temporary memory loss) induced by scopolamine, diazepam, and even alcohol. Possibly, its anti-inflammatory and antioxidant properties helped facilitate neurotransmitter function in the brain.

Active compounds in licorice that exert these effects are categorized as glycyrrhin and glycyrrhetic acid. Many other plant sterols (botanical compounds similar to human steroid hormones) contribute to its overall anti-inflammatory, antibacterial, and antiviral properties. In addition, the glycyrrhin and glycyrrhetic acids act as glucocorticoids in the human body. Remember that glucocorticoids are hormones made by the adrenal glands in response to pituitary prompting with ACTH. They have profound, long-lasting effects on energy metabolism in the body. Glucocorticoids deliver nutrients through the bloodstream to feed the different cells and tissues and organs of the body in times of stress. Cortisol, a classic glucocorticoid, has the overall effect of breaking down stored fats and proteins and carbohydrates to make these nutrients available for use as energy in the body. One of the issues with individuals afflicted with CFS is their reduced ability to produce adequate amounts of cortisol, especially in the morning when it should be at its maximum.[139,140] Licorice extends the longevity of cortisol action in the body and allows for more cortisol to be available in the morning. It seems to do so by suppressing the action of an enzyme 5-beta-reductase, thereby prolonging its effects, and fueling the glucocorticoid activity.[141] Together, its antiviral characteristics as well as its glucocorticoid-supporting actions make licorice an almost essential botanical for treatment of CFS.

Although no large clinical trials to date have tested the effects of licorice root on those with CFS, a number of studies elaborate on using artificial cortisol as treatment for CFS. One study of thirty-two individuals with CFS taking 5 to 10 mg of hydrocortisone (artificial cortisol medication) reported improvements in fatigue scores, some of which were similar to those reported by the "normal" population.[142] Another study of seventy individuals with CFS taking similar low-doses of hydrocortisone found improvement in wellness scores higher than placebo and outlasting placebo by several days.[143] Unfortunately, several participants experienced suppression of their adrenal gland function from using hydrocortisone in this experiment. The authors suggest that although some improvement was noted, this type of adrenal suppression "precludes its practical use for CFS." Perhaps the body interprets this administered cortisol as a reason to slow down its own natural synthesis of this hormone. While synthetic cortisol mimics the effects of the body's own cortisol, medicinal licorice root tends to prolong the lifetime of the cortisol already produced by the adrenal glands. In this way, it is less likely to suppress adrenal function while still enhancing the cortisol action in the body. Treatment with licorice root may be a superior alternative to hydrocortisone administration.

One very interesting case study points out the benefits of using licorice to treat an individual with CFS.[144] A fellow in Italy who was plagued with CFS for 20 years declared that his physical and mental stamina had returned to normal after taking licorice. Even his chronically swollen lymph nodes started to "go down." However, he did warn against using licorice in those with depression, as this condition tends to have the opposite hormonal picture with cortisol levels already being too high. In fact, licorice is not for everyone. Excessive consumption of licorice can cause symptoms of aldosterone excess such as headaches, fatigue, high blood pressure, water retention, leg swelling, and even heart attacks. These symptoms typically occur with the use of large doses of licorice, beyond what is normally recommended. Nevertheless, people who already suffer from high blood pressure, obesity, diabetes, or kidney, heart, or liver conditions should avoid licorice. This herb should also not be used by pregnant or breast-feeding women or by men with decreased libido or other sexual dysfunctions due to its hormonal influence.

Because herbs have medicinal properties, they can potentially interact with other herbs, medications, and supplements. Since licorice can induce some adverse effects if taken incorrectly, it is vital to consult a health-care provider in the field of botanical medicine before starting treatment with this herb. A practitioner who also has expertise in herbal medicines would be ideal for calculating effective and appropriate dosages for the individual, as well as for long-term monitoring of any potential consequences.

Appropriate dosage for most adults is 1 to 5 grams of dried root daily, boiled as a tea form. Other routes of therapy include using 2 to 5 mL of a licorice tincture or 250 to 500 mg of standardized extract containing 20 percent glycyrrhizinic acid. Any of these three approaches can be taken up to three times daily. Children should be given a fraction of the adult dose based on their weight divided by 150 lb (70 kg) for an adult. Usually, children can best consume licorice in the form of tea and liquid extracts, at about 1/3 of the typical dose given to adults. Use of any licorice product is not recommended for longer than 4 to 6 weeks.

Licorice dosages:

- Dried root: 1 to 5 grams as an infusion or decoction (boiled), three times daily

- Licorice 1:5 tincture: 2 to 5 mL, three times daily
- Standardized extract: 250 to 500 mg, three times daily, standardized to contain 20 percent glycyrrhizinic acid.

Withania somnifera (Ashwagandha)

Ashwagandha is also nicknamed the Indian ginseng. In Ayurvedic medicine it has been honored for thousands of years to be a daily rasayana, or antiaging therapy. Its Sanskrit name, which translates literally to "the strength of a horse," fits this herb well. Traditionally, ashwagandha has been revered as an adaptogen and immune modulator, nourishing and strengthening the inner reserve of the human body. It is a rejuvenative, a general tonic to the whole system, providing high levels of iron and amino acids such as glycine, valine, tyrosine, and alanine making it a very nutritive food as well as a medicinal herb.[145] It is known to reduce inflammation and calm down anxiety through its sedative effects. It has also been used for thousands of years to reduce stress, fever, pain, and high blood pressure. This panacea of an herb can treat asthma by relaxing the smooth muscles surrounding the airways into the lungs, allowing for improved breathing function. It can also support the function of the thyroid gland, enabling synthesis and release of thyroid hormones. By mimicking the effects of a neuropeptide called gamma-aminobutyric acid (GABA), it can lower anxiety and stress while also reducing convulsions in those with epilepsy.[146,147,148,149]

The root, which is its most medicinal part, contains active constituents including alkaloids (isopelletierine, anaferine), steroidal lactones (withanolides, withaferins), and saponins[148,149] but no nicotine as some researchers had previously thought.[145] These compounds also provide powerful antioxidant qualities. In fact, ashwagandha can restore glutathione levels that are depleted from fatigue.[2] It can also normalize catalase, glutathione reductase, and superoxide dismutase, all enzymes that become depleted with oxidative damage.[150] It can also significantly reduce lipid peroxidation from oxidative stress, improving overall antioxidant status.[151]

As a general immune tonic, ashwagandha's withanolides and sitoindosides activate macrophages and lysosomal enzymes to engulf foreign disease-causing agents.[149] The root contains compounds which act to fight off bacteria, fungus, ameba, parasites, and worms. These compounds also promote one pathway of the immune system, Th1, which boosts macrophage activity.[152] It can be used in oncology as an adjunct treatment to increase bone marrow cell and white blood cell count in people with cancer.[146] It can also reduce cyclophosphamide-induced immunosuppression and leucopenia.[146,153]

Antistress and adaptogenic actions of ashwagandha merit attention for the ability to treat people with CFS. On a physiological level, this botanical medicine can suppress stress-induced increases of dopamine receptors in the corpus striatum of the brain.[145] It can moderate the stress-induced increases of cortisol, blood urea nitrogen, and blood lactic acid.[149] As a glucocorticoid-like herb containing plant sterols, its actions are similar to those of licorice. It can extend the lifespan of cortisol in the body while controlling excessive increases of cortisol from stress.

Ashwagandha may be able to reverse and reduce severity of all the physiological changes due to long-term stress: increased blood glucose, glucose intolerance, gastric ulcers, male sexual dysfunction, cognitive deficits, immunosuppression, and mental depression.[154] In addition, it can promote the rebuilding of injured neural tissues associated with symptoms of memory loss. When neurons in the brain wither away, or atrophy, ashwagandha can induce significant regeneration of both axons and dendrites (ends of neurons) while reconstructing their synapses (connections).[155] This makes it an important medicinal herb to consider with conditions affecting mental function.

Ashwagandha is a relatively safe herb for regular consumption. Thousands of years of daily use as a rejuvenating formula in India provide credit to its use today. Generally, an appropriate adult dose would be 1 to 6 grams daily of the whole herb in capsule or tea form.[145] The tea is prepared by boiling ashwagandha roots in water for 15 minutes and cooled. The usual dose is three cups daily. Fresh plant liquid extracts or tinctures can be taken in dosages of 2 to 4 mL up to four times per day. Children should take no more than 1/3 of the adult dosage listed here.

Ashwagandha dosages:

- 1 to 6 grams of whole dried herb in tea or capsule form daily
- 2 to 4 mL of fresh plant liquid extract or tincture up to four times daily.

Ocimum sanctum (Holy Basil)

Holy Basil is a garden plant, a member of the same family as that of the more commonly used basil in Asian and Italian cuisine. Holy basil differs in that it is treated with great reverence in Indian culture and in Ayurvedic medicine, hence its name. This plant is commonly cultivated near temples and in homes for its ability to purify and sanctify its surroundings. Its leaves contain high levels of flavonoids, imparting an antioxidant quality, as well as many other active constituents. It is known to be a powerful anti-inflammatory herb, reducing pain and swelling by blocking certain pathways that lead to the inflammatory state.[156] In several ancient systems of medicine including Ayurveda, Greek, Roman, Siddha, and Unani, holy basil has a vast number of therapeutic uses for the heart, blood, respiratory system, liver and digestive system, and skin disorders. This herb has even been used traditionally for fevers, ear aches, ringworm, and other infectious diseases.[157] It is also more recently getting a lot more attention in research for its efficacy in treating diabetes, reducing cholesterol and triglycerides, and protecting against heart disease.[158,159,160]

As a medicinal plant rich in flavonoids, holy basil provides a solid dose of antioxidants. It can protect against chromosome damage caused by radiation. This plant seems to increase the body's production of glutathione and other enzymes responsible for reducing oxidative stress.[161] In doing so, holy basil can be protective to the brain and enhances mental performance.[162]

Holy basil has cognitive enhancement as well as adaptogenic benefits. It can ameliorate age-related memory loss and mental problems. A study of mice found that holy basil protected and reversed the cognitive decline associated with use of diazepam, barbiturates, and alcohol.[163] It seems to also work as an antistress remedy, a central nervous system stimulant that does not exaggerate the stress response. One group of researchers compared holy basil with desipramine, an antidepressant drug, in its ability to reduce stress and mood decline.[164] In another experiment, holy basil reduced the effects of chronic stress by controlling rises in blood sugar, depression, cognitive dysfunction, and immune suppression. The effects of holy basil on stress resistance were comparable to some of the ginsengs.[165] While there are no current studies on holy basil's use in CFS, it makes a good fit for its stress-resistant, antioxidant, and cognitive qualities. It can be safely taken on a regular basis at an adult dosage of 100 to 300 mg daily of the dried herb, or 3 to 4 tsp of the fresh herb brewed as a tea daily.

Holy basil dosages:

- 100 to 300 mg dried herb daily
- 3 to 4 tsp of fresh herb brewed in 8 ounces of tea daily.

MOOD AND MENTAL ENHANCING BOTANICALS

CFS is characterized by cognitive dysfunction including neurological impairment. Brain scans show lack of blood perfusion to areas of the brain that seems to reflect some kind of organic problem. Reduced blood flow may explain some of the mental impairment associated with CFS, leading to symptoms such as memory loss, depression, slow cognitive functioning, and others. There are a couple of key botanical medicines useful for improving blood circulation to the brain and helping to support mental clarity along with emotional well-being. Many of the herbs in the adaptogen category also support cognitive function and they are discussed in detail in the section on "Adaptogenic Botanicals." A couple of botanicals stand out as mood and mental enhancing medicines for those with CFS.

Hypericum perforatum (St John's Wort)

St. John's wort grows wild in dry soils and disturbed areas all throughout North America and parts of Europe. This plant is characterized by bright yellow flowers and leaves with tiny translucent dots that let the sunlight through. Its use dates back 2,000 years ago in ancient Greece for treatment of "nervous disorders" such as insomnia, depression, and anxiety. Other European uses included topical liniment applications of the deep red oils and resins from the flowers for bruises, sores, sprains, swellings, and wounds. Several Native American nations prescribed this herb internally for reducing fever, controlling bloody diarrhea, and bringing on menstruation. Historically, St John's wort has also been used to treat stomach aches, colic, urinary tract infections, and even uterine cramping. As a powerful antiviral medicine, it was rubbed on venereal sores and ulcers and given to counteract the effects of snake bites.[26]

Although roots and leaves have been chewed for medicine historically, the most applicable parts used today are the flowers. St John's wort is popularly known for its ability to lift the mood. In fact, it is one of the most commonly purchased herbal products in the United States for this reason. It is also one of the best-researched plant medicines at this time. Active constituents are hypericin and hyperforin, as well as melatonin to a lesser degree.[166,167] Many chemical constituents appear to contribute to the antidepressant action, and dozens of research studies have confirmed the role of St John's wort in elevating mood, often comparing its efficacy to that of Prozac.[168,169,170] These chemical compounds regulate the effects of neurotransmitters in the brain by limiting the reuptake (or depletion) of serotonin, dopamine, and norepinephrine.[171,172,173] Primarily, the effects on serotonin are responsible for its antidepressant activity.[173] This plant medicine acts like many antidepressant pharmaceutical medications as a selective serotonin receptor antagonist.[174] This means that it prolongs the time that serotonin (and other neurotransmitters in the brain) can exert its effects. Longevity of serotonin for most people leads to improved mood and mental outlook.

While the antidepressant effects have gained the most press, the lesser known benefit of these influences on neurotransmission is that it can cause cortisol stimulation in a dose-dependent manner.[175] As CFS is characterized by lower ranges of cortisol, this stimulation might be beneficial for reducing the fatigue. Also, hypericin and other compounds can reduce uptake (depletion) of gamma-butyric acid (GABA) and L-glutamate,[176,177] two neurotransmitters vital for the feelings of calm and relaxation. Preliminary research suggests that this plant medicine may be able to reduce anxiety as well as depression.[178]

St John's wort can effectively treat mild to moderate depression with fewer side effects than most prescriptive antidepressant medications. However, it is not appropriate for treating those with severe depression, complete inability to maintain daily functions, bipolar disorder, or suicidal ideation. It is important to consult with a physician if the depression is more serious. While side effects are not very common, they can include hives and skin rash, and sensitivity of the skin to sunlight. Therefore, it is important to avoid overexposure to the sun and tanning booths while taking this herbal medicine. Other adverse reactions may show up as restlessness, headache, dry mouth, and dizziness. In addition, St John's wort tends to interact with medications used during surgery and needs to be discontinued about 1 week prior to any surgery. Because St John's wort speeds up the metabolism of many pharmaceutical medications, it is strongly advised to check with a practitioner before starting on this herb if also taking medications. Individuals with mild-moderate depression need to consult a health-care provider trained in pharmacology as well as natural medicine before tapering off conventional antidepressant medications and switching to St John's wort. Women who are pregnant, trying to become pregnant, or breastfeeding should completely avoid this herb. While this herb is safe for many who have "the blues" from time to time, it is always best to get appropriate medical advice before starting St John's wort.

The usual dose for mild depression and mood disorders is 300 mg of dry herb in capsules or tablets (standardized to 0.3% hypericin extract), three times per day, with meals. St. John's wort is available in time-release capsules. It generally takes 3 to 4 weeks to notice changes.

St John's wort dosages:

- Liquid extract (1:1): forty to sixty drops, two times per day
- Tea: Pour one cup of boiling water over 2 to 4 tsp of dried St. John's wort and steep for 10 minutes. Drink up to three cups per day for 4 to 6 weeks
- Oil or cream: To treat inflammation, as in wounds, burns or hemorrhoids, an oil-based preparation of St. John's wort can be applied topically

Gingko biloba (Gingko)

Gingko trees are among the oldest living tree species in the world, as they can live for thousands of years. The history of its medicinal uses dates back to 2,600 B.C. when it was described in the first Chinese medicine pharmacopoeia for treating asthma and bronchitis.[179] While historically the fruit was used, in modern times the leaves are considered the most medicinal part of the plant, often in a standardized extract form for potency. This plant is famous as a best-seller in France, Germany, and even the United States. The volume of research around the medicinal properties of this plant is quite immense. In Europe and the United States, ginkgo supplements are among the best-selling herbal medications and it consistently ranks as a top medicine prescribed in France and Germany. In these countries, gingko is taken for its antioxidant value and for preventing age-related memory decline. In fact, the National Center for Complementary and Alternative Medicine (NCCAM) conducted a 5-year study of 3,000 people aged 75 finding that 240 mg gingko extract daily may prevent dementia or Alzheimer's disease.[180]

Active constituents include two groups of chemicals: terpenoids and a variety of flavonoids such as rutin, quercetin, and even proanthocyanidins. Each of these compounds can have instrinsic pharmacological properties in and of themselves, however, they seem to work synergistically to produce more potent effects as a team.[181,182] Perhaps one of the most popular uses of gingko is for its free radical scavenging actions of its many flavonoid components.[183,184,185,186,187] Not only do these flavonoids protect against oxidative damage to cell membranes but they also reduce this damage to red blood cells, an issue common to those with CFS.[188] Gingko seems to have an affinity for nervous tissue and can also protect against oxidative damage and injury to neurons.[186,189]

In addition to its use as an antioxidant, gingko may benefit people with CFS through its anti-inflammatory and circulatory actions. It is known to promote blood flow in capillaries to the brain, eyes, ears, and other areas where small blood vessels often become easily obstructed. This action happens because gingko can relax smooth muscles, allowing small blood vessels to dilate, while simultaneously making the blood less viscous so that it can travel through the vessels more effortlessly.[190,191] This improved circulation of blood to the brain may counteract some of the issues of low perfusion common in CFS.

While gingko is generally safe to take, it should not be consumed in very large doses. A particular chemical, gingkotoxin, which is present in higher concentrations in the seeds than the leaves, can potentially induce seizures in excessive amounts.[192,193] This is usually not an issue with gingko extracts using leaves.[194] Other side effects are rare but may include headaches, gastrointestinal upset, dizziness, and skin reactions. Since gingko can decrease platelet aggregation in the blood, it should not be used in combination with any other blood-thinning agents such as aspirin and nonsteroidal anti-inflammatory agents such as ibuprofen. Excessive use of gingko in combination with these pharmaceutical drugs can lead to a higher risk of easy bleeding and prolonged bleeding time. For this reason, any gingko preparation should be discontinued at least 36 hours prior to surgery due to potential risk for bleeding out. Women who are pregnant and breastfeeding should avoid taking any gingko supplements.

For cognitive improvement, daily dosages of 120 to 750 mg of the herb with 24 to 32 percent flavone gingkolides and 6 to 12 percent terpenoids (triterpene lactones) are typical.[195,196,197] Results may take 4 to 6 weeks to manifest but tend to accumulate after that time, thus likely requiring smaller dosages later.

Gingko dosages:

- 120 to 750 mg of herb with 24 to 32 percent gingkolides and 6 to 12 percent terpenoids daily for at least 4 to 6 weeks

SUMMARY OF BOTANICAL MEDICINES FOR CFS

With any multifactorial, complex condition like CFS, the treatment strategy needs to be comprehensive enough to embrace the subtleties and nuances of the individual affected by the condition. Botanical medicines are among the most ideal forms of therapy to achieve this unique effect. Each of the herbs described acts as a panacea with its many healing properties and varieties of uses in both traditional and modern medicine. Research studies may, for the time being, necessitate a simpler, clearer understanding of each herb's active constituents and their biochemical qualities. In clinical practice, however, the reality of these plant medicines is that they each provide a wealth and abundance of healing properties. Even though they have been neatly categorized by their primary benefits for people with CFS, we can see that each botanical prescription overlaps among the different categories, multitasking beyond our reductionistic views. For example, a plant that is classified as an adaptogen may also provide high levels of antioxidants, modulate the immune system, improve cognitive function, and support a sense of mood elevation and well-being. In addition to the already-mentioned health benefits, these plants also provide plenty of vitamins, minerals, oils, and other nutrients needed for creating vitality. Table 9.1 reviews the botanical medicines mentioned in this chapter, along with their healing properties and dosages.

Table 9.1. Summary of Botanical Medicines for Chronic Fatigue Syndrome

Botanical Name	Therapeutic Dosages	Medicinal Properties
St John's wort	• Liquid extract (1:1): forty to sixty drops, two times per day • Tea: Pour one cup of boiling water over 2–4 tsp of dried St. John's wort and steep for 10 minutes. Drink up to three cups per day for 4–6 weeks	Antidepressant, antioxidant, antiviral
Bilberry and Blueberry	• 20–60 mg (up to 320 mg) with 25% anthocyanidin content daily • 5–10 grams or 1–2 tsp of mashed or dried berries per cup of boiling water	Antioxidant, antifatigue
Elderberry	• 15 mL elderberry juice or extract up to four times daily during acute infections	Antioxidant, immune-enhancing
Grape	• 360–720 mg of grape seed extract containing 40–80% proanthocyanidins or 95% OPC	Antioxidant
Green tea	• 1–2 tsp of dried green tea herb per cup of boiling water, drunk three to four times daily • 300–400 mg standardized extract with 240–320 mg polyphenol content daily	Antioxidant, immune-enhancing
Amla fruit	• 1–3 tsp of Chyawanprash jam daily	Antioxidant, immune-enhancing, antiinflammatory, rejuvenative
Echinacea	• Freeze-dried extract 100–300 mg capsules containing 4% phenolics three times daily • Liquid herb juice twenty drops every hour during active infections • 2–3 mL three times daily of the tincture (preserved in alcohol) • 1–2 grams of dried root or herb in 8 ounces of boiling water drunk as tea three times daily • Always take a weeklong break from Echinacea treatment every 8 weeks before resuming	Antiviral, antibacterial, immuneenhancing
Astragalus	• Decoction (strong boiled tea): 3–6 grams of dried root per 12 ounces of water, three times per day • Fluid extract (1:1) in 25% ethanol: 2–4 mL three times a day	Antioxidant, antiviral, antibacterial, immune-enhancing

(Continued)

Table 9.1. (*Continued*)

Botanical Name	Therapeutic Dosages	Medicinal Properties
	• Powdered root: 500–1,000 mg three or four times per day • Powdered extract (solid): 100–150 mg of a product standardized to 0.5% 4-hydroxy-3-methoxy isoflavone. *Note*: this chemical is used only as a manufacturing marker, not as a guarantee of potency or effectiveness • Ointment: 10% astragalus applied to surface of wound. Do not apply to open wound without your doctor's supervision • Tincture (1:5) in 30% ethanol: 3–5 mL three times a day	
Reishi and Shiitake mushrooms	Reishi dosages: • $1\frac{1}{2}$ grams up to 9 grams daily of crude dried herb • $1\frac{1}{2}$ grams dried herb powder daily • 1 mL of alcohol-preserved tincture daily Shiitake dosages: • 75–150 mg of alcohol preserved tincture three times daily for up to 8 weeks at a time	Immune-enhancing
Cat's claw	• 20–150 mg dry standardized extract up to three times daily • $\frac{1}{4}$ to $\frac{1}{2}$ tsp of alcoholic tincture of herb up to three times daily • 1–10 grams of dry herb boiled in 8 ounces of water, up to 3 cups of tea daily	Immune-enhancing, antiinflammatory
Panax ginseng	• 15 mg standardized ginsenosides up to three times daily for 3 weeks on, 2 weeks off, 3 weeks on again	Antimicrobial, immune-enhancing, adaptogenic, antistress, antifatigue
Siberian ginseng, Eleuthrococcus	• Dried root: 2–4 grams in tea or capsules daily • Tincture (1:5): $\frac{1}{2}$ to 1 tsp three times daily • Fluid extract (1:1): 2–4 mL • Solid extract of dry, powdered root (20:1 or standardized to contain greater than 1% eleuthroside E): 100–200 mg twice daily	Rejuvenative, adaptogenic, immune-enhancing, antifatigue, extends the activity of cortisol

Table 9.1. (*Continued*)

Botanical Name	Therapeutic Dosages	Medicinal Properties
	• All dosages should be taken 3 weeks on, 2 weeks off, then 3 weeks on again!	
Rhodiola	• 50–100 mg of standardized herb capsules or aqueous extract (with 3% rosavins and 1% salidrosides) twice daily for 4 weeks, then 1 week rest before resuming treatment	Adaptogenic, stress-resistant, antioxidant, cognitive and memory enhancing, immune-enhancing, anti-inflammatory
Licorice	• Dried root: 1–5 grams as an infusion or decoction (boiled), three times daily • Licorice 1:5 tincture: 2–5 mL, three times daily • Standardized extract: 250–500 mg, three times daily, standardized to contain 20% glycyrrhizinic acid	Antiviral, adaptogenic, antioxidant, antiinflammatory, enhances cortisol activity
Ashwagandha	• 1–6 grams of whole dried herb in tea or capsule form daily • 2–4 mL of fresh plant liquid extract or tincture up to four times daily	Adaptogenic, rejuvenative, nutritive, sedative, relaxant, antioxidant, immune tonic, neuroregenerative, enhances cortisol effects
Holy basil	• 100–300 mg dried herb daily • 3–4 tsp of fresh herb brewed in 8 ounces of tea daily	Antioxidant, adaptogenic, anti-inflammatory, cognitive-enhancing, stress-resistant
Gingko	• 120–750 mg of herb with 24–32% gingkolides and 6–12% terpenoids daily for at least 4–6 weeks	Antioxidant, neuroprotective, supports blood flow to the brain, improves cognitive function, anti-inflammatory

For CFS sufferers, it is best to start by including some of these plants into the everyday diet, and rounding out the diet by supplementing these botanicals in the forms of teas, extracts, or capsules. It is best to start with one or two of the botanicals that seem to match the individual's symptoms for a few weeks before jumping to others. While these plant medicines are generally safe for most individuals, it is strongly recommended to seek guidance from a health-care practitioner trained in herbal medicines to customize the treatment plans and monitor progress with these medicines.

Resources

CFS ORGANIZATIONS & RESEARCH

American Association of CFS
The International Association for CFS/ME
27 N. Wacker Drive Suite 416
Chicago, IL 60606
847-258-7248
www.aacfs.org

Centers for Disease Control and Prevention
1600 Clifton Rd, Atlanta, GA 30333
(800) 311-3435
www.cdc.gov/cfs

CFIDS Association of America
PO Box 220398
Charlotte, NC 28222-0398
704.365.2343
www.cfids.org

PubMed online research
www.nlm.nih.gov/medlineplus/chronicfatiguesyndrome.html
www.niaid.nih.gov/factsheets/cfs.html
www.nlm.nih.gov/nccam/camonpubmed.html

ALTERNATIVE MEDICINE ORGANIZATIONS & INSTITUTES

Association of Accredited Naturopathic Medical Colleges
4435 Wisconsin Ave NW, Suite 403
Washington DC 20016
202.237.8150
www.aanmc.org

American Association of Naturopathic Physicians
4435 Wisconsin Ave NW, Suite 403
Washington DC 20016
866.538.2267
www.naturopathic.org

American Association of Oriental Medicine
PO Box 162340
Sacramento, CA 95816
866.455.7999
www.aaom.org

American College for the Advancement of Medicine
24411 Ridge Route Ste 115
Laguna Hills, CA 92653
949.309.3520
www.acamnet.org

American Holistic Medical Association
PO Box 2016
Edmonds, WA 98020
425.967.0737
www.holisticmedicine.org

The Ayurvedic Institute
PO Box 23445, Albuqueque NM 87192-1445
505.291.9698
www.ayurveda.com

Homeopathic Academy of Naturopathic Physicians
PO Box 126, Redmond WA 98073
www.hanp.net

North American Society of Homeopaths
PO Box 450039
Sunrise FL 33345-0039
206.720.7000
www.homeopathy.org

National Ayurvedic Medical Association
620 Cabrillo Ave, Santa Cruz CA 95065
800.669.8914
www.ayurveda-nama.org

National Commission for Certification of Acupuncture and Oriental Medicine
76 South Laura St, Suite 1290, Jacksonville FL 32202
904.598.1005
www.nccaom.org

References

CHAPTER 1

1. Wessely S. Old wine in new bottles: Neurasthenia and "ME." *Psychol Med* 1990;20:35–53.

2. Byrne E. Idiopathic chronic fatigue and myalgia syndrome (myalgic encephalomyelitis): Some thoughts on nomenclature and aetiology. *Med J Aust* 1988;148:80–82.

3. Wessely S, Hotopf M, Sharpe M. *Chronic fatigue and its syndromes.* Oxford: Oxford University Press, 1998.

4. Fukuda K, Straus SE, Hickie I, Sharpe MC, Dobbins JG, Komaroff A. The chronic fatigue syndrome: A comprehensive approach to its definition and study. *Ann Intern Med* 1994;121:953–959.

5. Carruthers BM, Jain AK, DeMeirleir KI. Myalgic encephalomyelitis/chronic fatigue syndrome: Clinical working case definition, diagnostic and treatment protocols. *J Chronic Fatigue Syndr* 2003;11:7–115.

6. Fukuda K Complete text of revised case definition. *Ann Intern Med* December 15, 1994;121:953–959.

7. Fukuda K, Gantz NM. Management strategies for chronic fatigue syndrome. *Fed Pract* 1995;12:12–27.

8. Komaroff AL, Fagioli LR, Geiger AM, Doolittle TH, Lee J, Kornish RJ, Gleit MA, Guerriero RT. An examination of the working case definition of chronic fatigue syndrome. *Am J Med* 1996;100:56–64.

9. Vercoulen JH, Swanink CM, Zitman FG, Vreden SG, Hoofs MP, Fennis JF, Galama JM, van der Meer JW, Bleijenberg G. A randomized, double-blind, placebo-controlled study of fluoxetine in chronic fatigue syndrome. *Lancet* 1996;347:858–861.

10. Kroenke K, Wood DR, Mangelsdorff AD, Meier NJ, Powell JB. Chronic fatigue in primary care. Prevalence, patient characteristics, and outcome. *JAMA* 1988;206:929–934.

11. Bates DW, Schmitt W, Buchwald D, Ware NC, Lee J, Thoyer E, Kornish RJ, Komaroff AL. Prevalence of fatigue and chronic fatigue syndrome in a primary care practice. *Arch Intern Med* 1993;153:2759–2765.

12. Price RK, North CS, Wessely S, Fraser VJ. Estimating the prevalence of chronic fatigue syndrome and associated symptoms in the community. *Public Health Rep* 1992;107:514–522.

13. Walker EA, Katon WJ, Jemelka RP. Psychiatric disorders and medical care utilization among people in the general population who report fatigue. *J Gen Intern Med* 1993;8:436–440.

14. Gunn WJ, Connell DB, Randall B. Epidemiology of chronic fatigue syndrome: The centers for disease control study. *Ciba Found Symp* 1993;173:83–93.

15. Reyes M, Gary HE Jr, Dobbins JG, Randall B, Steele L, Fukuda K, Holmes GP, Connell DG, Mawle AC, Schmid DS, Stewart JA, Schonberger LB, Gunn WJ, Reeves WC. Surveillance for chronic fatigue syndrome–four U.S. Cities, September 1989 through August 1993. *MMWR CDC Surveill Summ* February 21, 1997;46(2):1–13.

16. Reyes M, Nisenbaum R, Hoaglin DC, Unger ER, Emmons C, Randall B, Stewart JA, Abbey S, Jones JF, Gantz N, Minden S, Reeves WC. Prevalence and incidence of chronic fatigue syndrome in Wichita, Kansas. *Arch Intern Med* July 14, 2003;163(13):1530–1536.

17. Steele L, Dobbins JG, Fukuda K, Reyes M, Randall B, Koppelman M, Reeves WC. The epidemiology of chronic fatigue in San Francisco. *Am J Med* September 28, 1998;105(3A):83S–90S.

18. Buchwald D, Umali P, Umali J, Kith P, Pearlman T, Komaroff AL. Chronic fatigue and the chronic fatigue syndrome: Prevalence in a Pacific Northwest health care system. *Ann Intern Med* July 15, 1995;123(2):81–88.

19. Lindal E, Stefansson JG, Bergmann S. The prevalence of chronic fatigue syndrome in Iceland—a national comparison by gender drawing on four different criteria. *Nord J Psychiatry* 2002;56(4):273–277.

20. Jones JF, Nisenbaum R, Solomon L, Reyes M, Reeves WC. Chronic fatigue syndrome and other fatiguing illnesses in adolescents: A population-based study. *J Adolesc Health* July 2004;35(1):34–40.

21. Prins JB, vanderMeer JWM, Bleijenberg G. Chronic fatigue syndrome. *Lancet* 2006;367:346–355.

22. Bierl C, Nisenbaum R, Hoaglin DC, Randall B, Jones AB, Unger ER, Reeves WC. Regional distribution of fatiguing illnesses in the United States: A pilot study. *Popul Health Metr* Febuary 4, 2004;2(1):1.

23. Jason LA, Richman JA, Rademaker AW, Jordan KM, Plioplys AV, Taylor RR, McCready W, Huang CF, Plioplys S. A community-based study of chronic fatigue syndrome. *Arch Intern Med* 1999;159:2129–2137.

24. Hoogveld S, Prins J, deJong L. Personality characteristics and the chronic fatigue syndrome: A review of the literature. *Gedragstherapie* 2001;34:275–305.

25. Hickie I, Kirk K, Martin N. Unique genetic and environmental determinants of prolonged fatigue: A twin study. *Psychol Med* 1999;29:259–268.

26. White PD. What causes chronic fatigue syndrome? *BMJ* 2004;329:928–929.

27. Jason LA, Fennell PA, Taylor RR, eds. *Handbook of chronic fatigue syndrome*. Hoboken, NJ: John Wiley & Sons, 2003:108–123.

28. Hatcher S, House A. Life events, difficulties and dilemmas in the onset of chronic fatigue syndrome: A case-control study. *Psychol Med* 2003;33:1185–1192.

29. Moss-Morris R, Petrie KJ, Weinman J. Functioning in chronic fatigue syndrome: Do illness perceptions play a regulatory role? *Br J Health Psychol* 1996;1:15–25.

30. Petrie K, Moss-Morris R, Weinman J. The impact of catastrophic beliefs on functioning in chronic fatigue syndrome? *Psychol Med* 2001;31:107–114.

31. Cleare AJ. The neuroendocrinology of chronic fatigue syndrome. *Endocr Rev* 2003;24:236–252.

32. Kelley KW, Bluthé RM, Dantzer R, Zhou JH, Shen WH, Johnson RW, Broussard SR. Cytokine-induced sickness behavior. *Brain Behav Immun* 2003;17:S112–S118.

33. de Lange FP, Kalkman JS, Bleijenberg G, Hagoort P, van der Werf SP, van der Meer JW, Toni I. Neural correlates of the chronic fatigue syndrome: An fMRI study. *Brain* 2004;127:1948–1957.

34. Afari N, van de Meer J, Bleijenberg G, Buchwald D. Chronic fatigue syndrome in practice. *Psychiatr Ann* 2005;35:350–360.

35. Steinberg P, McNutt BE, Marshall P, Schenck C, Lurie N, Pheley A, Peterson PK. Double-blind placebo-controlled study of the efficacy of oral terfenadine in the treatment of chronic fatigue syndrome. *J Allergy Clin Immunol* January 1996;97(1 Pt 1):119–126.

36. Lloyd AR, Hickie I, Brockman A, Hickie C, Wilson A, Dwyer J, Wakefield D. Immunologic and psychologic therapy for patients with chronic fatigue syndrome: A double-blind, placebo-controlled trial. *Am J Med* February 1993;94(2):197–203.

37. Vollmer-Conna U, Hickie I, Hadzi-Pavlovic D, Tymms K, Wakefield D, Dwyer J, Lloyd A. Intravenous immunoglobulin is ineffective in the treatment of patients with chronic fatigue syndrome. *Am J Med* July 1997;103(1):38–43.

38. Iwakami E, Arashima Y, Kato K, Komiya T, Matsukawa Y, Ikeda T, Arakawa Y, Oshida S. Treatment of chronic fatigue syndrome with antibiotics: Pilot study assessing the involvement of Coxiella burnetii infection. *Intern Med* December 2005;44(12):1258–1263.

CHAPTER 2

1. Manningham R. *The symptoms, nature, causes and cure of the febricula or little fever: Commonly called the nervous or hysteric fever; The fever on the spirits; vapours, hypo, or spleen*, 2nd edn. London: J Robinson, 1750:52–53.

2. Beard G. Neurasthenia, or nervous exhaustion. *Boston Med Surg J* 1869;3:217–220.

3. DaCosta JM. On irritable heart: A clinical study of a form of functional cardiac disorder and its consequence. *Am J Med Sci* 1871;121:17–52.

4. Wood P. Aetiology of da costa's syndrome. *BMJ* 1941;845–851.

5. Buchwald D, Cheney PR, Peterson DL, Henry B, Wormsley SB, Geiger A, Ablashi DV, Salahuddin SZ, Saxinger C, Biddle R. A chronic illness characterized by fatigue, neurologic and immunologic disorders, and active human herpes virus type 6 infection. *Ann Intern Med* 1992;116:103–113.

6. Evans AC. Brucellosis in the United States. *Am J Public Health* 1947;37:139–151.

7. Jones JF, Ray CG, Minnich LL, Hicks MJ, Kibler R, Lucas DO. Evidence for active Epstein-Barr virus infection in patients with persistent, unexplained illnesses: Elevated anti-early antigen antibodies. *Ann Intern Med* 1985;102:1–7.

8. Holmes GP, Kaplan JE, Stewart JA, Hunt B, Pinsky PF, Schonberger LB. A cluster of patients with a chronic mononucleosis-like syndrome. Is Epstein-Barr virus the cause? *JAMA* 1987;260:2297–2298.

9. Stewart DE, Raskin J. Psychiatric assessment of patients with "20th-century disease" ("total allergy syndrome"). *Can Med Assoc J* 1985;133:1001–1006.

10. Lloyd AR, Wakefield D, Boughton CR, Dwyer JM. Immunological abnormalities in the chronic fatigue syndrome. *Med J Aust* August 7, 1989;151(3):122–124.

11. Zhang Q, Zhou XD, Denny T, Ottenweller JE, Lange G, LaManca JJ, Lavietes MH, Pollet C, Gause WC, Natelson BH. Changes in immune parameters seen in Gulf War veterans but not in civilians with chronic fatigue syndrome. *Clin Diagn Lab Immunol* January 1999;6(1):6–13.

12. Gupta S, Vayuvegula B. A comprehensive immunological analysis in chronic fatigue syndrome. *Scand J Immunol* March 1991;33(3):319–327.

13. Barker E, Fujimura SF, Fadem MB, Landay AL, Levy JA. Immunologic abnormalities associated with chronic fatigue syndrome. *Clin Infect Dis* January 1994;18(Suppl 1):S136–S141.

14. Tirelli U, Marotta G, Improta S, Pinto A. Immunological abnormalities in patients with chronic fatigue syndrome. *Scand J Immunol* December 1994;40(6):601–608.

15. Klimas NG, Salvato FR, Morgan R, Fletcher MA. Immunologic abnormalities in chronic fatigue syndrome. *J Clin Microbiol* July 1990;28(6):1403–1410.

16. Ogawa M, Nishiura T, Yoshimura M, Horikawa Y, Yoshida H, Okajima Y, Matsumura I, Ishikawa J, Nakao H, Tomiyama, Y, Kanayama Y, Kanakura Y, Matsuzawa Y. Decreased nitric oxide-mediated natural killer cell activation in chronic fatigue syndrome. *Eur J Clin Invest* November 1998;28(11):937–943.

17. Racciatti D, Vecchiet J, Ceccomancini A, Ricci F, Pizzigallo E. Chronic fatigue syndrome following a toxic exposure. *Sci Total Environ* April 10, 2001;270(1–3):27–31.

18. Maher KJ, Klimas NG, Fletcher MA. Chronic fatigue syndrome is associated with diminished intracellular perforin. *Clin Exp Immunol* December 2005;142(3):505–511.

19. Peakman M, Deale A, Field R, Mahalingam M, Wessely S. Clinical improvement in chronic fatigue syndrome is not associated with lymphocyte subsets of function or activation. *Clin Immunol Immunopathol* January 1997;82(1):83–91.

20. Linde A, Andersson B, Svenson SB, Ahrne H, Carlsson M, Forsberg P, Hugo H, Karstorp A, Lenkei R, Lindwall A. Serum levels of lymphokines and soluble cellular receptors in primary Epstein-Barr virus infection and in patients with chronic fatigue syndrome. *J Infect Dis* July 1992;165(6):994–1000.

21. Cohen J & Powderly WG. *Infectious diseases*, 2nd edn., 2004 Mosby, An Imprint of Elsevier. Written by Nelson M Gantz.

22. Kerr JR, Tyrrell DA. Cytokines in parvovirus B19 infection as an aid to understanding chronic fatigue syndrome. *Curr Pain Headache Rep* October 2003;7(5):333–341.

23. Patarca R. Cytokines and chronic fatigue syndrome. *Ann N Y Acad Sci* March 2001;933:185–200.

24. Patarca R, Klimas NG, Lugtendorf S, Antoni M, Fletcher MA. Dysregulated expression of tumor necrosis factor in chronic fatigue syndrome: Interrelations with cellular sources and patterns of soluble immune mediator expression. *Clin Infect Dis* January 1994;18(Suppl 1):S147–S153.

25. Landay AL, Jessop C, Lennette ET, Levy JA. Chronic fatigue syndrome: clinical condition associated with immune activation. *Lancet.* September 21, 1991;338(8769):707–712.

26. Hooper R. Waking up to chronic fatigue. *New Sci* 2006;190:2552.

27. Lloyd AR, Wakefield D, Hickie I. Immunity and the pathophysiology of chronic fatigue syndrome. *Ciba Found Symp* 1993;173:176–187; discussion 187–192.

28. Prieto J, Subira ML, Castilla A, Serrano M. Naloxone-reversible monocyte dysfunction in patients with chronic fatigue syndrome. *Scand J Immunol* July 1989;30(1):13–20.

29. Siegel SD, Antoni M, Fletcher MA, Maher K, Segota MC, Klimas N. Impaired natural immunity, cognitive dysfunction, and physical symptoms in patients with chronic fatigue syndrome: Preliminary evidence for a subgroup? *J Psychosom Res* June 2006;60(6):559–566.

30. Young E. Brain holds the key to chronic fatigue. *New Sci* 2006;189:2542.

31. Komaroff AL. Is human herpesvirus-6 a trigger for chronic fatigue syndrome? *J Clin Virol* December 2006;37(Suppl 1):S39–S46.

32. Manian FA. Simultaneous measurement of antibodies to Epstein-Barr virus, human herpesvirus 6, herpes simplex virus types 1 and 2, and 14 enteroviruses in chronic fatigue syndrome: Is there evidence of activation of a nonspecific polyclonal immune response? *Clin Infect Dis* September 1994;19(3):448–453.

33. Jones JF, Ray CG, Minnich LL, Hicks MJ, Kibler R, Lucas DO. Evidence for active Epstein-Barr virus infection in patients with persistent, unexplained illnesses: Elevated anti-early antigen antibodies. *Ann Intern Med* 1985;102:1–7.

34. Straus SE, Tosato G, Armstrong G, Lawley T, Preble OT, Henle W, Davey R, Pearson G, Epstein J, Brus I. Persisting illness and fatigue in adults with evidence of Epstein-Barr virus infection. *Ann Intern Med* 1985;102:7–16.

35. Matthews DA, Lane TJ, Manu P. Antibodies to Epstein-Barr virus in patients with chronic fatigue. *South Med J* July 1991;84(7):832–840.

36. Kawai K, Kawai A. Studies on the relationship between chronic fatigue syndrome and Epstein-Barr virus in Japan. *Intern Med* March 1992;31(3):313–318.

37. Buchwald D, Sullivan JL, Komaroff AL. Frequency of chronic active Epstein-Barr virus infection in a general medical practice. *JAMA* 1987;257:2303–2307.

38. Gold D, Bowden R, Sixbey J, Riggs R, Katon WJ, Ashley R, Obrigewitch RM, Corey L. Chronic fatigue. A prospective clinical and virologic study. *JAMA* July 4, 1990;264(1):48–53.

39. Hellinger WC, Smith TF, Van Scoy RE, Spitzer PG, Forgacs P, Edson RS. Chronic fatigue syndrome and the diagnostic utility of antibody to Epstein-Barr virus early antigen. *JAMA* August 19, 1988;260(7):971–973.

40. Mawle AC, Nisenbaum R, Dobbins JG, Gary HE Jr, Stewart JA, Reyes M, Steele L, Schmid DS, Reeves WC. Seroepidemiology of chronic fatigue syndrome: A case-control study. *Clin Infect Dis* 1995;21:1386–1389.

41. Yousef GE, Bell EJ, Mann GF, Murugesan V, Smith DG, McCartney RA, Mowbray JF. Chronic enterovirus infection in patients with postviral fatigue syndrome. *Lancet* 1988;i:146–150.

42. Archard LC, Bowles NE, Behan PO, Bell EJ, Doyle D. Postviral fatigue syndrome: Persistence of enterovirus RNA in muscle and elevated creatine kinase. *J Roy Soc Med* 1988;81:326–329.

43. Swanink CM, Melchers WJ, van der Meer JW, Vercoulen JH, Bleijenberg G, Fennis JF, Galama JM. Enteroviruses and the chronic fatigue syndrome. *Clin Infect Dis* 1994;19:860–864.

44. DeFreitas E. Retroviral sequence related to human T-lymphocytic virus type II in patients with CFIDS. *Proc Natl Acad Sci U.S.A* 1991;88,2922–2926.

45. Imboden JB, Canter A, Cluff LE, Trever RW. Brucellosis. III. Psychological aspects of delayed convalescence. *Arch Intern Med* 1959;103:406–414.

46. Imboden JB, Canter A, Cluff LE. Convalescence from influenza. A study of the psychological and clinical determinants. *Arch Intern Med* 1961;108:393–399.

47. Dinerman H, Steere AC. Lyme disease associated with fibromyalgia. *Ann Intern Med* 1992;11:281–285.

48. Straus SE, Dale JK, Wright R, Metcalfe DD. Allergy and the chronic fatigue syndrome. *J Allergy Clin Immunol* May 1988;81(5 Pt 1):791–795.

49. Marcusson JA, Lindh G, Evengard B. Chronic fatigue syndrome and nickel allergy. *Contact Dermatitis* May 1999;40(5):269–272.

50. Ferre YL, Cardona DV, Cadahia GA. Prevalence of atopy in chronic fatigue syndrome. *Allergol Immunopathol (Madr)* January-February 2005;33(1):42–47.

51. Conti F, Magrini L, Priori R, Valesini G, Bonini S. Eosinophil cationic protein serum levels and allergy in chronic fatigue syndrome. *Allergy* February 1996;51(2):124–127.

52. Bellanti JA, Sabra A, Castro HJ, Chavez JR, Malka-Rais J, de Inocencio JM. Are attention deficit hyperactivity disorder and chronic fatigue syndrome allergy related? What is fibromyalgia? *Allergy Asthma Proc* January-February 2005;26(1):19–28.

53. Manu P, Matthews DA, Lane TJ. Food intolerance in patients with chronic fatigue. *Int J Eat Disord* March 1993;13(2):203–209.

54. Logan AC, Wong C. Chronic fatigue syndrome: Oxidative stress and dietary modifications. *Altern Med Rev* October 2001;6(5):450–459.

55. Jacobsen MB, Aukrust P, Kittang E, Müller F, Ueland T, Bratlie J, Bjerkeli V, Vatn MH. Relation between food provocation and systemic immune activation in patients with food intolerance. *Lancet* July 29, 2000;356(9227):400–401.

56. Emms TM, Robers TK, Butt HL, et al. *Food intolerance in chronic fatigue syndrome*. Abstract #15 presented at the American Association for Chronic Fatigue Syndrome conference. Seattle, WA: January 2001.

57. Gibson SL, Gibson RG. A multidimensional treatment plan for chronic fatigue syndrome. *J Nutr Environ Med* 1999;9:47–54.

58. Dunstan RH, Donohoe M, Taylor W, Roberts TK, Murdoch RN, Watkins JA, McGregor NR. A preliminary investigation of chlorinated hydrocarbons and chronic fatigue syndrome. *Med J Aust* September 18, 1995;163(6):294–297.

59. Fulle S, Mecocci P, Fano G, Vecchiet I, Vecchini A, Racciotti D, Cherubini A, Pizzigallo E, Vecchiet L, Senin U, Beal MF. Specific oxidative alterations in vastus lateralis muscle of patients with the diagnosis of chronic fatigue syndrome. *Free Radic Biol Med* December 15, 2000;29(12):1252–1259.

60. Vecchiet J, Cipollone F, Falasca K, Mezzetti A, Pizzigallo E, Bucciarelli T, De Laurentis S, Affaitati G, De Cesare D, Giamberardino MA. Relationship between musculoskeletal symptoms and blood markers of oxidative stress in patients with chronic fatigue syndrome. *Neurosci Lett* January 2, 2003;335(3):151–154.

61. Richards RS, Roberts TK, McGregor NR, Dunstan RH, Butt HL. Blood parameters indicative of oxidative stress are associated with symptom expression in chronic fatigue syndrome. *Redox Rep* 2000;5(1):35–41.

62. Richards RS, Wang L, Jelinek H. Erythrocyte oxidative damage in chronic fatigue syndrome. *Arch Med Res* January 2007;38(1):94–98.

63. Manuel y Keenoy B, Moorkens G, Vertommen J, De Leeuw I. Antioxidant status and lipoprotein peroxidation in chronic fatigue syndrome. *Life Sci* March 16, 2001;68(17):2037–2049.

64. Jammes Y, Steinberg JG, Mambrini O, Bregeon F, Delliaux S. Chronic fatigue syndrome: Assessment of increased oxidative stress and altered muscle excitability in response to incremental exercise. *J Intern Med* March 2005;257(3):299–310.

65. Maes M, Mihaylova I, Leunis JC. Chronic fatigue syndrome is accompanied by an IgM-related immune response directed against neopitopes formed by oxidative or nitrosative damage to lipids and proteins. *Neuro Endocrinol Lett* October 2006;27(5):615–621.

66. Maes M, Mihaylova I, De Ruyter M. Lower serum zinc in Chronic Fatigue Syndrome (CFS): Relationships to immune dysfunctions and relevance for the oxidative stress status in CFS. *J Affect Disord* February 2006;90(2–3):141–147.

67. Pall ML. Elevated, sustained peroxynitrite levels as the cause of chronic fatigue syndrome. *Med Hypothesis* 2002 Jan;54(1):115–125.

68. Pall ML, Satterlee JD. Elevated nitric oxide/peroxynitrite mechanism for the common etiology of multiple chemical sensitivity, chronic fatigue syndrome, and posttraumatic stress disorder. *Ann N Y Acad Sci* March 2001;933:323–329.

69. Radi R, Rodriguez M, Castro L, Telleri R. Inhibition of mitochondrial electron transport by peroxynitrite. *Arch Biochem Biophys* January 1994;308(1):89–95.

70. Kennedy G, Spence VA, McLaren M, Hill A, Underwood C, Belch JJ. Oxidative stress levels are raised in chronic fatigue syndrome and are associated with clinical symptoms. *Free Radic Biol Med* September 1, 2005;39(5):584–589.

71. Natelson BH, Cohen JM, Brassloff I, Lee HJ. A controlled study of brain magnetic resonance imaging in patients with the chronic fatigue syndrome. *J Neurol Sci* December 15, 1993;120(2):213–217.

72. Lange G, DeLuca J, Maldjian JA, Lee H, Tiersky LA, Natelson BH. Brain MRI abnormalities exist in a subset of patients with chronic fatigue syndrome. *J Neurol Sci* December 1, 1999;171(1):3–7.

73. Greco A, Tannock C, Brostoff J, Costa DC. Brain MR in chronic fatigue syndrome. *AJNR Am J Neuroradiol* August 1997;18(7):1265–1269.

74. Schwartz RB, Komaroff AL, Garada BM, Gleit M, Doolittle TH, Bates DW, Vasile RG, Holman BL. SPECT imaging of the brain: Comparison of findings in patients with chronic fatigue syndrome, AIDS dementia complex, and major unipolar depression. *Am J Roentgenol* April 1994;162(4):943–951.

75. Costa DC, Tannock C, Brostoff J. Brainstem perfusion is impaired in chronic fatigue syndrome. *QJM* November 1995;88(11):767–773.

76. Ichise M, Salit IE, Abbey SE, Chung DG, Gray B, Kirsh JC, Freedman M. Assessment of regional cerebral perfusion by 99Tcm-HMPAO SPECT in chronic fatigue syndrome. *Nucl Med Commun* October 1992;13(10):767–772.

77. Yoshiuchi K, Farkas J, Natelson B. Patients with chronic fatigue syndrome have reduced absolute cortical blood flow. *Clin Physiol Funct Imaging* March 2006;26(2):83–86.

78. Ash-Bernal R, Wall C 3rd, Komaroff AL, Bell D, Oas JG, Payman RN, Fagioli LR. Vestibular function test anomalies in patients with chronic fatigue syndrome. *Acta Otolaryngol* January 1995;115(1):9–17.

79. Saggini R, Pizzigallo E, Vecchiet J, Macellari V, Giacomozzi C. Alteration of spatial-temporal parameters of gait in chronic fatigue syndrome patients. *J Neurol Sci* January 21, 1998;154(1):18–25.

80. Boda WL, Natelson BH, Sisto SA, Tapp WN. Gait abnormalities in chronic fatigue syndrome. *J Neurol Sci* August 1995;131(2):156–161.

CHAPTER 3

1. Tintera JW. The hypoadrenocortical state and its management. *NY State J Med* 1955;55:1869–1876.

2. Demitrack MA, Dale JK, Straus SE, Laue L, Listwak SJ, Kruesi MJ, Chrousos GP, Gold PW. Evidence for impaired activation of the hypothalamic-pituitary-adrenal axis in patients with chronic fatigue syndrome. *J Clin Endocrinol Metab* December 1991;73(6):1224–1234.

3. Cleare AJ, Miell J, Heap E, Sookdeo S,Young L, Malhi GS, O'Keane V. Hypothalamo-pituitary-adrenal axis dysfunction in chronic fatigue syndrome, and the effects of low-dose hydrocortisone therapy. *J Clin Endocrinol Metab* August 2001;86(8):3545–3554.

4. Jerjes WK, Peters TJ, Taylor NF, Wood PJ, Wessely S, Cleare AJ. Diurnal excretion of urinary cortisol, cortisone, and cortisol metabolites in chronic fatigue syndrome. *J Psychosom Res* February 2006;60(2):145–153.

5. Gaab J, Huster D, Peisen R, Engert V, Schad T, Schurmeyer TH, Ehlert U. Low-dose dexamethasone suppression test in chronic fatigue syndrome and health. *Psychosom Med* March-April 2002;64(2):311–318.

6. Young AH, Sharpe M, Clements A, Dowling B, Hawton KE, Cowen PJ. Basal activity of the hypothalamic-pituitary-adrenal axis in patients with the chronic fatigue syndrome (neurasthenia). *Biol Psychiatry* February 1, 1998;43(3):236–237.

7. Roberts AD, Wessely S, Chalder T, Papadopoulos A, Cleare AJ. Salivary cortisol response to awakening in chronic fatigue syndrome. *Br J Psychiatry* February 2004;184:136–141.

8. Jerjes WK, Cleare AJ, Wessely S, Wood PJ, Taylor NF. Diurnal patterns of salivary cortisol and cortisone output in chronic fatigue syndrome. *J Affect Disord* August 2005;87(2–3):299–304.

9. McKenzie R, O'Fallon A, Dale J, Demitrack M, Sharma G, Deloria M, Garcia-Borreguero D, Blackwelder W, Straus SE. Low-dose hydrocortisone for treatment of chronic fatigue syndrome: A randomized controlled trial. *JAMA* September 23–30, 1998;280(12):1061–1066.

10. Peterson PK, Pheley A, Schroeppel J, Schenck C, Marshall P, Kind A, Haugland JM, Lambrecht LJ, Swan S, Goldsmith S. A preliminary placebo-controlled crossover trial of fludrocortisone for chronic fatigue syndrome. *Arch Intern Med* April 27, 1998;158(8):908–914.

11. Hudson M, Cleare AJ. The 1microg short Synacthen test in chronic fatigue syndrome. *Clin Endocrinol (Oxf)* November 1999;51(5):625–630.

12. Mommersteeg PM, Heijnen CJ, Verbraak MJ, van Doornen LJ. Clinical burnout is not reflected in the cortisol awakening response, the day-curve or the response to a low-dose dexamethasone suppression test. *Psychoneuroendocrinology* February 2006;31(2):216–225. Epub 2005 Sep 16.

13. Grossi G, Perski A, Ekstedt M, Johansson T, Lindstrom M, Holm K. The morning salivary cortisol response in burnout. *J Psychosom Res* August 2005;59(2):103–111.

14. Nicolson NA, van Diest R. Salivary cortisol patterns in vital exhaustion. *J Psychosom Res* November 2000;49(5):335–342.

15. Demitrack MA, Crofford LJ. Evidence for and pathophysiologic implications of hypothalamic-pituitary-adrenal axis dysregulation in fibromyalgia and chronic fatigue syndrome. *Ann N Y Acad Sci* May 1, 1998;840:684–697.

16. Demitrack MA, Dale JK, Straus SE, Laue L, Listwak SJ, Kruesi MJ, Chrousos GP, Gold PW. Evidence for impaired activation of the hypothalamic-pituitary-adrenal axis in patients with chronic fatigue syndrome. *J Clin Endocrinol Metab* December 1991;73(6):1224–1234.

17. Scott LV, Medbak S, Dinan TG. Blunted adrenocorticotropin and cortisol responses to corticotropin-releasing hormone stimulation in chronic fatigue syndrome. *Acta Psychiatr Scand* June 1998;97(6):450–457.

18. Di Giorgio A, Hudson M, Jerjes W, Cleare AJ. 24-hour pituitary and adrenal hormone profiles in chronic fatigue syndrome. *Psychosom Med* May-June 2005;67(3):433–440.

19. Gaab J, Huster D, Peisen R, Engert V, Heitz V, Schad T, Schurmeyer TH, Ehlert U. Hypothalamic-pituitary-adrenal axis reactivity in chronic fatigue syndrome and health under psychological, physiological, and pharmacological stimulation. *Psychosom Med* November-December 2002;64(6):951–962.

20. Gaab J, Engert V, Heitz V, Schad T, Schurmeyer TH, Ehlert U. Associations between neuroendocrine responses to the Insulin Tolerance Test and patient characteristics in chronic fatigue syndrome. *J Psychosom Res* April 2004;56(4):419–424.

21. Scott LV, Svec F, Dinan T. A preliminary study of dehydroepiandrosterone response to low-dose ACTH in chronic fatigue syndrome and in healthy subjects. *Psychiatry Res* December 4, 2000;97(1):21–28.

22. Cleare AJ, O'Keane V, Miell JP. Levels of DHEA and DHEAS and responses to CRH stimulation and hydrocortisone treatment in chronic fatigue syndrome. *Psychoneuroendocrinology* July 2004;29(6):724–732.

23. Scott LV, Medbak S, Dinan TG. Desmopressin augments pituitary-adrenal responsivity to corticotropin-releasing hormone in subjects with chronic fatigue syndrome and in healthy volunteers. *Biol Psychiatry* June 1, 1999;45(11):1447–1454.

24. Altemus M, Dale JK, Michelson D, Demitrack MA, Gold PW, Straus SE. Abnormalities in response to vasopressin infusion in chronic fatigue syndrome. *Psychoneuroendocrinology* February 2001;26(2):175–188.

25. Bennett AL, Mayes DM, Fagioli LR, Guerriero R, Komaroff AL. Somatomedin C (insulin-like growth factor I) levels in patients with chronic fatigue syndrome. *J Psychiatr Res.* January–February 1997;31(1):91–96.

26. Cleare AJ, Sookdeo SS, Jones J. Integrity of the growth hormone/insulin-like growth factor system is maintained in patients with chronic fatigue syndrome. *J Clin Endocrinol Metab* April 2000;85(4):1433–1439.

27. Buchwald D, Umali J, Stene M. Insulin-like growth factor-I (somatomedin C) levels in chronic fatigue syndrome and fibromyalgia. *J Rheumatol* April 1996;23(4):739–742.

28. Moorkens G, Berwaerts J, Wynants H, Abs R. Characterization of pituitary function with emphasis on GH secretion in the chronic fatigue syndrome. *Clin Endocrinol (Oxf)* July 2000;53(1):99–106.

29. Korszun A, Sackett-Lundeen L, Papadopoulos E, Brucksch C, Masterson L, Engelberg NC, Haus E, Demitrack MA, Crofford L. Melatonin levels in women with fibromyalgia and chronic fatigue syndrome. *J Rheumatol* December 1999;26(12):2675–2680.

30. Demitrack MA, Gold PW, Dale JK, Krahn DD, Kling MA, Straus SE. Plasma and cerebrospinal fluid monoamine metabolism in patients with chronic fatigue syndrome: Preliminary findings. *Biol Psychiatry* December 15, 1992;32(12):1065–1077.

31. Yatham LN, Morehouse RL, Chisholm BT, Haase DA, MacDonald DD, Marrie TJ. Neuroendocrine assessment of serotonin (5-HT) function in chronic fatigue syndrome. *Can J Psychiatry* March 1995;40(2):93–96.

32. Inder WJ, Prickett TC, Mulder RT. Normal opioid tone and hypothalamic-pituitary-adrenal axis function in chronic fatigue syndrome despite marked functional impairment. *Clin Endocrinol (Oxf)* March 2005;62(3):343–348.

33. Hatcher S, House A. Life events, difficulties and dilemmas in the onset of chronic fatigue syndrome: A case-control study. *Psychol Med* October 2003;33(7):1185–1192.

34. Theorell T, Blomkvist V, Lindh G, Evengard B. Critical life events, infections, and symptoms during the year preceding chronic fatigue syndrome (CFS): An examination of CFS patients and subjects with a nonspecific life crisis. *Psychosom Med* May-June 1999;61(3):304–310.

35. DeLuca J, Johnson SK, Ellis SP, Natelson BH. Cognitive functioning is impaired in patients with chronic fatigue syndrome devoid of psychiatric disease. *J Neurol Neurosurg Psychiatry*. February 1997;62(2):151–155.

36. DeLuca J, Johnson SK, Beldowicz D, Natelson BH. Neuropsychological impairments in chronic fatigue syndrome, multiple sclerosis, and depression. *J Neurol Neurosurg Psychiatry* January 1995;58(1):38–43.

37. Marcel B, Komaroff AL, Fagioli LR, Kornish RJ 2nd, Albert MS. Cognitive deficits in patients with chronic fatigue syndrome. *Biol Psychiatry* September 15, 1996;40(6):535–541.

38. Marshall PS, Watson D, Steinberg P, Cornblatt B, Peterson PK, Callies A, Schenck CH. An assessment of cognitive function and mood in chronic fatigue syndrome. *Biol Psychiatry* February 1, 1996;39(3):199–206.

39. Capuron L, Welberg L, Heim C, Wagner D, Solomon L, Papanicolaou DA, Craddock RC, Miller AH, Reeves WC. Cognitive dysfunction relates to subjective report of mental fatigue in patients with chronic fatigue syndrome. *Neuropsychopharmacology* August 2006;31(8):1777–1784. Epub 2006 Jan 4.

40. DeLuca J, Johnson SK, Natelson BH. Information processing efficiency in chronic fatigue syndrome and multiple sclerosis. *Arch Neurol* March 1993;50(3):301–304.

41. Michiels V, de Gucht V, Cluydts R, Fischler B. Attention and information processing efficiency in patients with Chronic Fatigue Syndrome. *J Clin Exp Neuropsychol* October 1999;21(5):709–729.

42. Joyce E, Blumenthal S, Wessely S. Memory, attention, and executive function in chronic fatigue syndrome. *J Neurol NeurosurgPsychiatry* May 1996;60(5):495–503.

43. Wearden AJ, Appleby L. Research on cognitive complaints and cognitive functioning in patients with chronic fatigue syndrome (CFS): What conclusions can we draw? *J Psychosom Res* September 1996;41(3):197–211.

44. Busichio K, Tiersky LA, Deluca J, Natelson BH. Neuropsychological deficits in patients with chronic fatigue syndrome. *J Int Neuropsychol Soc* March 2004;10(2):278–285.

45. Marshall PS, Forstot M, Callies A, Peterson PK, Schenck CH. Cognitive slowing and working memory difficulties in chronic fatigue syndrome. *Psychosom Med* January-February 1997;59(1):58–66.

46. Mahurin RK, Claypoole KH, Goldberg JH, Arguelles L, Ashton S, Buchwald D. Cognitive processing in monozygotic twins discordant for chronic fatigue syndrome. *Neuropsychology* April 2004;18(2):232–239.

47. Lane TJ, Manu P, Matthews DA. Depression and somatization in the chronic fatigue syndrome. *Am J Med* October 1991;91(4):335–344.

48. Michielsen HJ, Van Houdenhove B. Depression, attribution style and self-esteem in chronic fatigue syndrome and fibromyalgia patients: Is there a link? *Clin Rheumatol* April 2006;25(2):183–188.

49. Lane TJ, Manu P, Matthews DA. Depression and somatization in the chronic fatigue syndrome. *Am J Med* October 1991;91(4):335–344.

50. Taerk GS, Toner BB, Salit IE, Garfinkel PE, Ozersky S. Depression in patients with neuromyasthenia (benign myalgic encephalomyelitis). *Int J Psychiatry Med* 1987;13:49–52.

51. Kruesi MJP, Dale J, Straus S. Psychiatric diagnoses in patients who have chronic fatigue. *J Clin Psychiatry* 1989;50:53–56.

52. Wessely S, Chalder T, Hirsch S, Wallace P, Wright D. Psychological symptoms, somatic symptoms, and psychiatric disorder in chronic fatigue and chronic fatigue syndrome: A prospective study in the primary care setting. *Am J Psychiatry* August 1996;153(8):1050–1059.

53. Gur A, Cevik R, Nas K, Colpan L, Sarac S. Cortisol and hypothalamic-pituitary-gonadal axis hormones in follicular-phase women with fibromyalgia and chronic fatigue syndrome and effect of depressive symptoms on these hormones. *Arthritis Res Ther* 2004;6(3):R232–R238. Epub 2004 Mar 15.

CHAPTER 4

1. Komaroff AL, Fagioli LR, Geiger AM, Doolittle TH, Lee J, Kornish RJ, Gleit MA, Guerriero RT. An examination of the working case definition of chronic fatigue syndrome. *Am J Med* 1996;100:56–64.

2. Buchwald D, Goldenberg DL, Sullivan JL, Komaroff AL. The "chronic active Epstein-Barr virus infection" syndrome and primary fibromyalgia. *Arthritis Rheum* 1987 Oct;30(10):1132–6.

3. Bell D. *The doctor's guide to chronic fatigue syndrome: understanding, treating, and living with CFIDS*. Reading, Massachusetts, 1994.

4. Komaroff AL. Chronic fatigue syndromes: Relationship to chronic viral infections. *J Virol Methods* 1988;21:3–10.

5. Bates DW, Buchwald D, Lee J, Kith P, Doolittle T, Rutherford C, Churchill WH, Schur PH, Wener M, Wybenga D. Clinical laboratory test findings in patients with chronic fatigue syndrome. *Arch Intern Med* 1995;155:97–103.

6. Gow JW, Behan PO. Viruses and chronic fatigue syndrome. *J CFS* 1996;2:67–83.

7. Komaroff AL. The biology of chronic fatigue syndrome. *Am J Med* 2000;108:169–171.

8. Bell DS. Chronic fatigue syndrome update: Findings now point to CNS involvement. *Postgrad Med* 1994;96:73–81.

9. Ablashi DV, Eastman HB, Owen CB, Roman MM, Friedman J, Zabriskie JB, Peterson DL, Pearson GR, Whitman JE. Frequent HHV-6 reactivation in multiple sclerosis and chronic fatigue syndrome patients. *J Clin Virol* 2000;16:179–191.

10. Martin WJ, Zeng LC, Ahmed K, Roy M. Cytomegalovirus-related sequence in an atypical cytopathic virus repeatedly isolated from a patient with chronic fatigue syndrome. *American J Pathol* 1994;145:440–451.

11. Khan AS, Heneine WM, Chapman LE, Gary HE Jr, Woods TC, Folks TM, Schonberger LB. Assessment of a retrovirus sequence and other possible risk factors for the chronic fatigue syndrome in adults. *Ann Intern Med* 1993;118:241–245.

12. Heneine W, Woods TC, Sinha SD, Khan AS, Chapman LE, Schonberger LB, Folks TM. Lack of evidence for infection with known human and animal retroviruses in patients with chronic fatigue syndrome. *Clin Infect Dis* 1994;18:121–125.

13. Honda M, Kitamura K, Nakasone T, Fukushima Y, Matsuda S, Nishioka K, Matsuda J, Hashimoto N, Yamazaki S. Japanese patients with chronic fatigue syndrome are negative for known retrovirus infections. *Microbiol Immunol* 1993;37:779–784.

14. Gow JW, Behan WM, Simpson K, McGarry F, Keir S, Behan PO. Studies on enterovirus in patients with chronic fatigue syndrome. *Clin Infect Dis* 1994;18:S126–S129.

CHAPTER 5

1. Demitrack MA, Dale JK, Straus SE, Laue L, Listwak SJ, Kruesi MJ, Chrousos GP, Gold PW. Evidence for impaired activation of the hypothalamic-pituitary-adrenal axis in patients with chronic fatigue syndrome. *J Clin Endocrinol Metab* December 1991;73(6):1224–1234.

2. Roberts AD, Wessely S, Chalder T, Papadopoulos A, Cleare AJ. Salivary cortisol response to awakening in chronic fatigue syndrome. *Br J Psychiatry* February 2004;184:136–141.

3. Scott LV, Medbak S, Dinan TG. Blunted adrenocorticotropin and cortisol responses to corticotropin-releasing hormone stimulation in chronic fatigue syndrome. *Acta Psychiatr Scand* June 1998;97(6):450–457.

4. Di Giorgio A, Hudson M, Jerjes W, Cleare AJ. 24-hour pituitary and adrenal hormone profiles in chronic fatigue syndrome. *Psychosom Med* May-June 2005;67(3):433–440.

5. Gaab J, Hüster D, Peisen R, Engert V, Heitz V, Schad T, Schürmeyer TH, Ehlert U. Hypothalamic-pituitary-adrenal axis reactivity in chronic fatigue syndrome and health under psychological, physiological, and pharmacological stimulation. *Psychosom Med* November-December 2002;64(6):951–962.

6. Vining RF, McGinley RA. The measurement of hormones in saliva: Possibilities and pitfalls. *J Steroid Biochem* 1987;27:81–94.

7. Tunn S, Mollmann H, Barth J, Derendorf H, Krieg M. Simultaneous measurement of cortisol in serum and saliva after different forms of cortisol administration. *Clin Chem* 1992;38:1491–1494.

8. Peter JR, Walker RF, Riad-Fahmy D, Hall R. Salivary cortisol assays for assessing pituitary-adrenal reserve. *Clin Endocrinol (Oxf)* 1982;17:583–592.

9. Gozansky WS, Lynn JS, Laudenslager ML, Kohrt WM. Salivary cortisol determined by enzyme immunoassay is preferable to serum total cortisol for assessment of dynamic hypothalamic–pituitary–adrenal axis activity. *Clin Endocrinol (Oxf)*. September 2005;63(3):336–341.

10. Fitzgerald PA. Adrenal cortex physiology. In: Tierney LM Jr, McPhee J, Papadakis MA, eds. *Current medical diagnosis and treatment*. Los Altos, CA: MA Lange Publishers, 1995.

11. Straus SE, Dale JK, Wright R, Metcalfe DD. Allergy and the chronic fatigue syndrome. *J Allergy Clin Immunol* May 1988;81(5 Pt 1):791–795.

12. Conti F, Magrini L, Priori R, Valesini G, Bonini S. Eosinophil cationic protein serum levels and allergy in chronic fatigue syndrome. *Allergy* February 1996;51(2):124–127.

13. Bellanti JA, Sabra A, Castro HJ, Chavez JR, Malka-Rais J, de Inocencio JM. Are attention deficit hyperactivity disorder and chronic fatigue syndrome allergy related? What is fibromyalgia? *Allergy Asthma Proc* January-February 2005;26(1):19–28.

14. Manu P, Matthews DA, Lane TJ. Food intolerance in patients with chronic fatigue. *Int J Eat Disord* March 1993;13(2):203–209.

15. Jacobsen MB, Aukrust P, Kittang E, Müller F, Ueland T, Bratlie J, Bjerkeli V, Vatn MH. Relation between food provocation and systemic immune activation in patients with food intolerance. *Lancet* July 29, 2000;356(9227):400–401.

16. Gibson SL, Gibson RG. A multidimensional treatment plan for chronic fatigue syndrome. *J Nutr Environ Med* 1999;9:47–54.

17. Logan AC, Wong C. Chronic fatigue syndrome: oxidative stress and dietary modifications. *Altern Med Rev* October 2001;6(5):450–459.

18. Butkus SN, Mahan LK. Food allergies: immunological reactions to food. *J Am Diet Assoc* 1986;86:601–608.

19. Andre F, Andre C, Feknous M, Colin L, Cavagna S. Digestive permeability to different-sized molecules and to sodium cromoglycate in food allergy. *Allergy Proc* 1991;12:293–298.

20. Andre C, Andre F, Colin L, Cavagna S. Measurement of intestinal permeability to mannitol and lactulose as a means of diagnosing food allergy and evaluating therapeutic effectiveness of disodium cromoglycate. *Ann Allergy* 1987;59:127–130.

21. Hunter JO. Food allergy—or enterometabolic disorder? *Lancet* 1991;338:495–496.

22. Russel GW, Kilian M, Lamm ME. Biological activities of IgA. In: Mestecky J, Bienenstock J, Lamm M, Strober W, McGhee J, Mayer L, eds. *Mucosal immunology*. San Diego, CA: Academic Press, 2004:225–240.

23. Gleeson M, McDonald WA, Cripps AW, Pyne DB, Clancy RL, Fricker PA, Wlodarrczyk JH. Exercise, stress, and mucosal immunity in elite athletes. *Adv Mucosal Immunol* 1995;2:571–574.

CHAPTER 6

1. Whiting P, Bagnall AM, Sowden AJ, Cornell JE, Mulrow CD, Ramírez G. Interventions for the treatment and management of chronic fatigue syndrome: A systematic review. JAMA. 2001 Sep 19;286(11):1360–1368.

2. Bertolin Guillen JM, Bedate ViUar J. Therapeutic guidelines in chronic fatigue syndrome. *Icto Luso Esp Neurol Psiquiatr Cienc Afines* 1994:22:127–130.

3. Singh BB, Vinjamury SP, Singh VJ. *Chronic fatigue syndrome: Integrative medicine: A systematic approach*. New York, NY: McGraw-Hill, 2003.

4. Bodane C, Brownson K. The growing acceptance of complementary and alternative medicine. *Health Care Manag (Frederick)* March 2002;20(3):11–21.

5. Canadian College of Naturopathic Medicine: Annual Report. Toronto, 1999.

6. Smith MJ, Logan AC. Naturopathy. *Med Clin North Am* January 2002;86(1):173–184.

7. Dunne N, Benda W, Kim L, Mittman P, Barrett R, Snider P, Pizzorno J. Naturopathic medicine: What can patients expect? *J Fam Pract* December 2005;54(12):1067–1072.

8. Dunne-Boggs N, Mittman P. Naturopathic medicine is an emerging field in one of medicine's most dynamic eras. *Med Gen Med* 2004;6(1):35.

9. Drivdahl C, Miser W. The use of alternative health care by a family practice population. *J Am Board Fam Pract* 1998;11:193–199.

10. National Research Council, *Diet and health. Implications for reducing chronic disease risk*. Washington, DC: National Academy Press, 1989.

11. Gaby AR. Intravenous nutrient therapy: The "Myers' cocktail." *Altern Med Rev* October 2002;7(5):389–403.

12. Harakeh S, Jariwalla RJ, Pauling L. Suppression of human immunodeficiency virus replication by ascorbate in chronically and acutely infected cells. *Proc Natl Acad Sci USA* 1990;87:7245–7249.

13. Okayama H, Aikawa T, Okayama M, Sasaki H, Mue S, Takishima T. Bronchodilating effect of intravenous magnesium sulfate in bronchial asthma. *JAMA* 1987;257:1076–1078.

14. Pizzorno J, Murray M. *The textbook of natural medicine*. St Louis: Elsevier, 2006.

15. Kleijnen J, Knipschild P, terRiet G. Clinical trials of homeopathy. *BMJ* 1991;302:316–323.

16. Geraghty J. Homeopathic treatment of chronic fatigue syndrome: Three case studies using Jan Scholten's methodology. *Homeopathy* April 2002;91(2):99–105.

17. Gibson SLM, Gibson RG. A multidimensional treatment plan for chronic fatigue syndrome. *J Nutr Environ Med* 1999;9(1):47–54.

18. Weatherley-Jones E, Nicholl JP, Thomas KJ, Parry GJ, McKendrick MW, Green ST, Stanley PJ, Lynch SP. A randomised, controlled, triple-blind trial of the efficacy of homeopathic treatment for chronic fatigue syndrome. *J Psychosom Res* 2004;56:189–197.

19. Awdry R. "Homeopathy and chronic fatigue—the search for proof," International Journal of Alternative and Complementary Medicine, 1996;14:12–16.

20. Titus GW. Providing alternative health care: An ancient system for a modern age. *Adv Pact Nurs Q* 1995 Winter;1(3):19–28.

21. Mishra L, Singh BB, Dagenais S. Ayurveda: A historical perspective and principles of the traditional healthcare system in India. *Altern Ther Health Med* 2001;7:36–42.

22. Hankey A. Ayurvedic physiology and etiology: Ayurvedo Amritanaam. The doshas and their functioning in terms of contemporary biology and physical chemistry. *J Altern Complement Med* October 2001;7(5):567–574.

23. Vinjamury SP, Singh BB. Ayurvedic treatment of chronic fatigue syndrome–a case report. *Altern Ther Health Med* September–October 2005;11(5):76–78.

24. Khan S, Balick MJ. Therapeutic plants of Ayurveda: A review of selected clinical and other studies for 166 species. *J Altern Complement Med* October 2001;7(5):405–515.

25. Jain SK. Ethnobotany and research on medicinal plants in India. *Ciba Found Symp* 1994;185:153–164; discussion 164–168.

26. Tripathi YB. Molecular approach to ayurveda. *Indian J Exp Biol* May 2000;38(5):409–414.

27. Maoshing N. *The yellow emperor's classic of medicine: A new translation of the neijing suwen with commentary*, edn 1. Boston: Shambhala, 1995.

28. Unschuld PU. *Medicine in China: A history of ideas*. Berkeley: University of California Press, 1985.

29. Acupuncture. *Consensus Development Conference Statement. National Institutes of Health*. Online at http://consensus.nih.gov/cons/107/107_statement.htm.

30. Zhu Guang-wen. Self-composed bu gan yi qi tang in the treatment of 46 cases of chronic fatigue syndrome. *Zhe Jiang Zhong Yi Za Zhi* (Zhejiang Journal of Chinese Medicine) 2000;11:476.

31. Lin Y, Ly H, Bioteau A. Acupuncture In The Management Of Chronic Fatigue Syndrome In Adolescents: A Pilot Study at the Chronic Fatigue Syndrome Clinic at the Children's Hospital Boston. *Am J Chin Med*. 2005;33(1):151–156.

32. Flaws B, Sionneau P. *The treatment of modern western diseases with Chinese medicine*. Boulder, CO: Blue Poppy Press, 2001.

CHAPTER 7

1. Pizzorno J, Murray M. *The textbook of natural medicine*, 3rd edn. St Louis: Elsevier, 2006.

2. Marz R. *Medical nutrition from Marz*. Portland: Omni-Press, 1999.

3. National Research Council. *Diet and health. Implications for reducing chronic disease risk*. Washington, DC: National Academy Press, 1989.

4. Brown L, Rosner B, Willett WW, Sacks FM. Cholesterol-lowering effects of dietary fiber: a meta-analysis. *Am J Clin Nutr* 1999;69:30–42.

5. National Research Council (U.S.), Committee on Diet and Health. *Diet and health: Implications for reducing chronic disease risk.* Washington, DC: National Academy Press, 1989.

6. Segasothy M, Phillips PA. Vegetarian diet: panacea for modern lifestyle diseases? *QJM* 1999;92:531–544.

7. Licata AA, Bou E, Bartter FC, West F. Acute effects of dietary protein on calcium metabolism in patients with osteoporosis. *J Geron* 1981;36:14–19.

8. Bougnoux P. N-3 polyunsaturated fatty acids and cancer. *Curr Opin Clin Nutr Metab Care* 1999;2:121–126.

9. Bucher HC, Hengstler P, Schindler C, Meier G. N-3 polyunsaturated fatty acids in coronary heart disease: A meta-analysis of randomized controlled trials. *Am J Med* 2002;112:298–304.

10. Fraser GE. Nut consumption, lipids, and risk of a coronary event. *Clin Cardiol* 1999;22(Suppl):11–15.

11. Jiang R, Manson JE, Stampfer MJ, Liu S, Willett WC, Hu FB. Nut and peanut butter consumption and risk of type 2 diabetes in women. *JAMA* 2002;288:2554–2560.

12. Lastra Alarcon de la C, Barranco MD, Motilva V, Herrerias JM. Mediterranean diet and health: Biological importance of olive oil. *Curr Pharm Des* 2001;7:933–950.

13. Kleiner SM. Water: An essential but overlooked nutrient. *J Am Diet Assoc* 1999;99:200–206.

14. Hughes JR, Higgins ST, Bickel WK, Hunt WK, Fenwick JW, Gulliver SB, Mireault GC. Caffeine self-administration, withdrawal, and adverse effects among coffee drinkers. *Arch Gen Psych* 1991;48:611–617.

15. Estler CJ, Ammon HP, Herzog C. Swimming capacity of mice after prolonged treatment with psychostimulants. I. Effects of caffeine on swimming performance and cold stress. *Psychopharmacology* 1978;58:161–166.

16. Greden JF, Fontaine P, Lubetsky M, Chamberlin K. Anxiety and depression associated with caffeinism among psychiatric inpatients. *Am J Psychiatry* 1978;135:963–966.

17. Steinmetz KA, Potter JD. Vegetables, fruit, and cancer. II. Mechanisms. *Cancer Causes Control* 1991;2:427–442.

18. Steinmetz KA, Potter JD. Vegetables, fruit, and cancer prevention: A review. *J Am Diet Assoc* 1996;96:1027–1039.

19. Vecchia La C, Tavani A. Fruit and vegetables, and human cancer. *Eur J Cancer Prev* 1998;7:3–8.

20. Duyn Van MA, Pivonka E. Overview of the health benefits of fruit and vegetable consumption for the dietetics professional: Selected literature. *J Am Diet Assoc* 2000;100:1511–1521.

21. Jenkins DJ, Kendall CW, Augustin LS, Franceschi S, Hamidi M, Marchie A, Jenkins AL, Axelsen M. Glycemic index: Overview of implications in health and disease. *Am J Clin Nutr* 2002;76:266S–267S.

22. Willett W, Manson J, Liu S. Glycemic index, glycemic load, and risk of type 2 diabetes. *Am J Clin Nutr* 2002;76:274S–280S.

23. Liu S, Willett WC, Stampfer MJ, Hu FB, Franz M, Sampson L, Hennekens CH, Manson JE. A prospective study of dietary glycemic load, carbohydrate intake, and risk of coronary heart disease in US women. *Am J Clin Nutr* 2000;71:1455–1461.

24. Bingham SA. High-meat diets and cancer risk. *Proc Nutr Soc* 1999;58:243–248.

25. Segasothy M, Phillips PA. Vegetarian diet: Panacea for modern lifestyle diseases?. QJM 1999;92:531–544.

26. Zheng W, Gustafson DR, Sinha R, Cerhan JR, Moore D, Hong CP, Anderson KE, Kushi LH, Sellers TA, Folsom AR. Well-done meat intake and the risk of breast cancer. J Natl Cancer Inst 1998;90:1724–1729.

27. Baris D, Zahm SH. Epidemiology of lymphomas. Curr Opin Oncol 2000;12:383–394.

28. Blair A, Zahm SH. Agricultural exposures and cancer. Environ Health Perspect 1995;103(Suppl 8):205–208.

29. Mao Y, Hu J, Ugnat AM, White K. Non-Hodgkin's lymphoma and occupational exposure to chemicals in Canada. Canadian Cancer Registries Epidemiology Research Group. Ann Oncol 2000;11(Suppl 1):69–73.

30. Jaga K, Brosius D. Pesticide exposure: Human cancers on the horizon. Rev Environ Health 1999;14:39–50.

31. Lu C, Knutson DE, Fisker-Andersen J, Fenske RA. Biological monitoring survey of organophosphorus pesticide exposure among preschool children in the Seattle metropolitan area. Environ Health Perspect 2001;109(3):299–303.

32. Boris M, Mandel FS. Foods and additives are common causes of the attention deficit hyperactive disorder in children. Ann Allergy 1994;72:462–468.

33. Lessof MH. Reactions to food additives. Clin Exp Allergy 1995;25(Suppl 1):27–28.

34. Groten JP, Butler W, Feron VJ, Kozianowski G, Renwick AG, Walker R. An analysis of the possibility for health implications of joint actions and interactions between food additives. Regul Toxicol Pharmacol 2000;31:77–91.

35. Simon RA. Adverse reactions to food additives. Curr Allergy Asthma Rep 2003;3:62–66. These include substances such as preservatives, artificial colors, artificial flavorings, and acidifiers.

36. Fahrner H. Fasten als Therapie. Stuttgart, Hippokrates.

37. Michalsen A, Weidenhammer W, Melchart D. Short-term therapeutic fasting in the treatment of chronic pain and fatigue syndromeswell-being and side effects with and without mineral supplements. Forsch Komplementarmed Klass Naturheilkd August 2002;9(4):221–227.

38. Masuda A, Nakayama T, Yamanaka T, Hatsutanmaru K, Tei C. Cognitive behavioral therapy and fasting therapy for a patient with chronic fatigue syndrome. Intern Med November 2001;40(11):1158–1161.

39. Michalsen A, Schneider S, Rodenbeck A. The short-term effects of fasting on the neuroendocrine system in patients with chronic pain syndromes. Nutr Neurosci February 2003;6(1):11–19.

40. Farmer ME, Locke BZ, Mościcki EK, Dannenberg AL, Larson DB, Radloff LS. Physical activity and depressive symptoms: The NHANES 1 epidemiologic follow-up study. Am J Epidemiol 1988;1328:1340–1351.

41. Fiatarone MA, Morley JE, Bloom ET, Benton D, Solomon GF, Makinodan T. The effect of exercise on natural killer cell activity in young and old subjects. J Gerontol 1989;44:M37–M45.

42. Makinnon LT. Exercise and natural killer cells. What is their relationship? Sports Med 1989;7:141–149.

43. Fitzgerald L. Exercise and the immune system. Immunol Today 1988;9:337–339.

44. Sun XS, Xu Y, Xia YJ. Determination of E-rosette-forming lymphocytes in aged subjects with Taichiquan exercise. Int J Sport Med 1989;10:217–219.

45. Nijs J, Meeus M, De Meirleir K. Chronic musculoskeletal pain in chronic fatigue syndrome: Recent developments and therapeutic implications. *Man Ther* August 2006;11(3):187–191.

46. Friedberg F. Does graded activity increase activity? A case study of chronic fatigue syndrome. *J Behav Ther Exp Psychiatry* 2002;33:203–215.

47. Wallman KE, Morton AR, Goodman C, Grove R, Guilfoyle AM. Randomised controlled trial of graded exercise in chronic fatigue syndrome. *Med J Aust* 2004;180:444–448.

48. Glass JM, Lyden AK, Petzke F, Stein P, Whalen G, Ambrose K, Chrousos G, Clauw DJ. The effect of brief exercise cessation on pain, fatigue, and mood symptom development in healthy, fit individuals. *J Psychosom Res* October 2004;57(4):391–398.

49. Soderlund A, Malterud K. Why did I get chronic fatigue syndrome? A qualitative interview study of causal attributions in women patients. *Scand J Prim Health Care* December 2005;23(4):242–247.

50. Turp E. Coping successfully with chronic fatigue. *Health Couns Psychother J* January 2006;6(1):22–25.

51. Prins JB, Bos E, Huibers MJ, Servaes P, van der Werf SP, van der Meer JW, Bleijenberg G. Social support and the persistence of complaints in chronic fatigue syndrome. *Psychother Psychosom* 2004;73:174–182.

52. Ax S, Gregg VH, Jones D. Chronic fatigue syndrome: Sufferers' evaluation of medical support. *J R Soc Med* May 1997;90(5):250–254.

CHAPTER 8

1. Singh A, Garg V, Gupta S, Kulkarni SK. Role of antioxidants in chronic fatigue syndrome in mice. *Indian J Exp Biol* November 2002;40(11):1240–1244.

2. Singh A, Naidu PS, Gupta S, Kulkarni SK. Effect of natural and synthetic antioxidants in a mouse model of chronic fatigue syndrome. *J Med Food* Winter 2002;5(4):211–220.

3. Manuel y, Keenoy B, Moorkens G, Vertommen J, De Leeuw I. Antioxidant status and lipoprotein peroxidation in chronic fatigue syndrome. *Life Sci* March 16, 2001;68(17):2037–2049.

4. Ockerman P. Antioxidant treatment of chronic fatigue syndrome. *Clin Pract Altern Med* 2000;1:88–91.

5. Maes M, Mihaylova I, De Ruyter M. Lower serum zinc in Chronic Fatigue Syndrome (CFS): Relationships to immune dysfunctions and relevance for the oxidative stress status in CFS. *J Affect Disord* February 2006;90(2-3):141–147. Epub 2005 Dec 9.

6. Grant JE, Veldee MS, Buchwald D. Analysis of dietary intake and selected nutrient concentrations in patients with chronic fatigue syndrome. *J Am Diet Assoc* 1996;96:383–386.

7. Jessop, Carol. Reported in the Fibromyalgia Network Newsletter compendium #2, October 1990–January 1992.

8. Odeh M. The role of zinc in acquired immunodeficiency syndrome. *J Intern Med* 1992;231:463–469.

9. Krotkiewski M, Gudmundsson M, Backstrom P, Mandroukas K. Zinc and muscle strength and endurance. *Acta Physiol Scand* 1982;116:309–311.

10. Packer L, Witt EH, Tritschler HJ. Alpha-Lipoic acid as a biological antioxidant. *Free Radic Biol Med* 1995;19:227–250.

11. Anon. Alpha-lipoic acid. *Altern Med Rev* 1998;3:308–310.

12. Biewenga GP, Haenen GR, Bast A. The pharmacology of the antioxidant lipoic acid. *Gen Pharmacol* 1997;29:315–331.

13. Packer L, Witt EH, Tritschler HJ. Alpha-Lipoic acid as a biological antioxidant. *Free Radic Biol Med* 1995;19:227–250.

14. Packer L, Tritschler HJ, Wessel K. Neuroprotection by the metabolic antioxidant alpha-lipoic acid. *Free Radic Biol Med* 1997;22:359–378.

15. Fuchs J, Schöfer H, Milbradt R, Freisleben HJ, Buhl R, Siems W, Grune T. Studies on lipoate effects on blood redox state in human immunodeficiency virus infected patients. *Arzneimittelforschung* 1993;43:1359–1362.

16. Lomaestro BM, Malone M. Glutathione in health and disease: Pharmacotherapeutic issues. *Ann Pharmacother* 1995;29:1263–1273.

17. Kelly GS. Clinical applications of N-acetylcysteine. *Altern Med Rev* 1998;3:114–127.

18. De Rosa SC, Zaretsky MD, Dubs JG, Roederer M, Anderson M, Green A, Mitra D, Watanabe N, Nakamura H, Tjioe I, Deresinski SC, Moore WA, Ela SW, Parks D, Herzenberg LA, Herzenberg LA. N-acetylcysteine replenishes glutathione in HIV infection. *Eur J Clin Invest* 2000;30:915–929.

19. Arthur JR. The glutathione peroxidases. *Cell Mol Life Sci* 2000;57:1825–1835.

20. Fleshner NE, Kucuk O. Antioxidant dietary supplements: Rationale and current status as chemopreventive agents for prostate cancer. *Urology* 2001;57:90–94.

21. Food and Nutrition Board, Institute of Medicine. *Dietary reference intakes for vitamin C, vitamin E, selenium, and carotenoids*. Washington, DC: National Academy Press, 2000.

22. Jiang Q, Christen S, Shigenaga MK, Ames BN. Gamma-tocopherol, the major form of vitamin E in the US diet, deserves more attention. *Am J Clin Nutr* 2001;74:714–722.

23. Ravaglia G, Forti P, Maioli F, Bastagli L, Facchini A, Mariani E, Savarino L, Sassi S, Cucinotta D, Lenaz G. Effect of micronutrient status on natural killer cell immune function in healthy free-living subjects aged >/=90 y. *Am J Clin Nutr* 2000;71:590–598.

24. Levine M, Rumsey SC, Daruwala R, Park JB, Wang Y. Criteria and recommendations for vitamin C intake. *JAMA* 1999;281:1415–1423.

25. Johnston CS, Thompson LL, Vitamin C. Status of an outpatient population. *J Am Coll Nutr* 1998;17:366–370.

26. Padayatty SJ, Levine M. New insights into the physiology and pharmacology of vitamin C. *CMAJ* 2001;164:353–355.

27. Hodges RE, Hood J, Canham JE, Sauberlich HE, Baker EM. Clinical manifestations of ascorbic acid deficiency in man. *Am J Clin Nutr* 1971;24:432–443.

28. Kinsman RA, Hood J. Some behavioral effects of ascorbic acid deficiency. *Am J Clin Nutr* 1971;24:455–464.

29. Gerster H. The role of vitamin C in athletic performance. *J Am Coll Nutr* 1989;8:636–643.

30. Heseker H, Kubler W, Pudel V, Westenhoffer J. Psychological disorders as early symptoms of a mild-to-moderate vitamin deficiency. *Ann N Y Acad Sci* 1992;669:352–357.

31. Anderson R. Ascorbate-mediated stimulation of neutrophil motility and lymphocyte transformation by inhibition of the peroxidase/H2O2/ halide system in vitro and in vivo. *Am J Clin Nutr* 1981;34:1906–1911.

32. Anderson R, Oosthuizen R, Maritz R, Theron A, Van Rensburg AJ. The effects of increasing weekly doses of ascorbate on certain cellular and humoral immune functions in normal volunteers. *Am J Clin Nutr* 1980;33:71–76.

33. Prinz W, Bortz R, Bregin B, Hersch M. The effect of ascorbic acid supplementation on some parameters of the human immunological defense system. *Int J Vitam Nutr Res* 1977;47:248–257.

34. Vallance S. Relationships between ascorbic acid and serum proteins of the immune system. *Br Med J* 1977;2:437–438.

35. Leibovitz B, Siegel BV. Ascorbic acid and the immune response. *Adv Exp Med Biol* 1981;135:1–25.

36. Roitt I. Immune processes can be influenced by neuroendocrine factors. *Essential immunology*. 8th edn Oxford-Blackwell Scientific Publications, London, Edinburgh, Boston 1994:210.

37. Kodama M, Kodama T. Murakami M. The value of the dehydroepiandrosterone-annexed vitamin C infusion treatment in the clinical control of chronic fatigue syndrome (CFS). I. A Pilot study of the new vitamin C infusion treatment with a volunteer CFS patient. *In Vivo* November-December 1996;10(6):575–584.

38. Kodama M, Kodama T. The clinical course of interstitial pneumonia alias chronic fatigue syndrome under the control of megadose vitamin C infusion system with dehydroepiandrosterone-cortisol annex. *Int J Mol Med* January 2005;15(1):109–116.

39. Manuel y, Keenoy B, Moorkens G, Vertommen J. Magnesium status and parameters of the oxidant-antioxidant balance in patients with chronic fatigue: Effects of supplementation with magnesium. *J Am Coll Nutr* June 2000;19(3):374–382.

40. Cox IM, Campbell MJ, Dowson D. Red blood cell magnesium and chronic fatigue syndrome. *Lancet* 1991;337:757–760.

41. Howard JM, Davies S, Hunnisett A. Magnesium and chronic fatigue syndrome. *Lancet* 1992;340:426.

42. Pizzorno J, Murray M. *The textbook of natural medicine*, 3rd edn. St Louis: Elsevier, 2006.

43. Ahlborg H, Ekelund LG, Nilsson CG. Effect of potassium-magnesium aspartate on the capacity for prolonged exercise in man. *Acta Physiol Scand* 1968;74:238–245.

44. Friedlander HS. Fatigue as a presenting symptom: management in general practice. *Curr Ther Res* 1962;4:441–449.

45. Shaw DL Jr, Chesney MA, Tullis IF. Agersborg HP. Management of fatigue: A physiologic approach. *Am J Med Sci* 1962;243:758–769.

46. Gaby AR. Intravenous nutrient therapy: The "Myers' cocktail." *Altern Med Rev* October 2002;7(5):389–403.

47. Gullestad L, Oystein Dolva L, Birkeland K, Falch D, Fagertun H, Kjekshus J. Oral versus intravenous magnesium supplementation in patients with magnesium deficiency. *Magnes Trace Elem* 1991;10:11–16.

48. Lindberg JS, Zobitz MM, Poindexter JR, Pak CY. Magnesium bioavailability from magnesium citrate and magnesium oxide. *J Am Coll Nutr* 1990;9:48–45.

49. Tapiero H, Couvreur GN, Tew KD. Polyunsaturated fatty acids (PUFAs) and eicosanoids in human health and pathologies. *Biomed Pharmacother* July 2002;56 no. 5:215–222.

50. Calder PC. N-3 polyunsaturated fatty acids, inflammation and immunity: Pouring oil on troubled waters or another fishy tale? *Nutr Res* 2001;21:309–341.

51. Mori TA, Burke V, Puddey IB, Watts GF, O'Neal DN, Best JD, Beilin LJ. Purified eicosapentaenoic and docosahexaenoic acids have differential effects on serum lipids and lipoproteins, LDL particle size, glucose, and insulin in mildly hyperlipidemic men. *Am J Clin Nutr* 2000;71:1085–1094.

52. Woodman RJ, Mori TA, Burke V, Puddey IB, Watts GF, Beilin LJ. Effects of purified eicosapentaenoic and docosahexaenoic acids on glycemic control, blood pressure, and serum lipids in type 2 diabetic patients with treated hypertension. *Am J Clin Nutr* 2002;76:1007–1015.

53. Nemets B, Stahl Z, Belmaker RH. Addition of omega-3 fatty acid to maintenance medication treatment for recurrent unipolar depressive disorder. *Am J Psychiatry* March 2002;159(3):477–479.

54. Erkkila AT, Lehto S, Pyorala K, Uusitupa MI. n-3 Fatty acids and 5-y risks of death and cardiovascular disease events in patients with coronary artery disease. *Am J Clin Nutr* July 2003;78(1):65–71.

55. Pischon T, Hankinson SE, Hotamisligil GS, Rifai N, Willett WC, Rimm EB. Habitual dietary intake of n-3 and n-6 fatty acids in relation to inflammatory markers among US men and women. *Circulation* July 15, 2003;108(2):155–160. Epub 2003 Jun 23.

56. Conquer JA, Holub BJ. Supplementation with an algae source of docosahexaenoic acid increases (n-3) fatty acid status and alters selected risk factors for heart disease in vegetarian subjects. *J Nutr* 1996;126:3032–3039.

57. Wainwright P. Nutrition and behaviour: The role of n-3 fatty acids in cognitive function. *Br J Nutr* 2000;83:337–339.

58. Gibson RA. Long-chain polyunsaturated fatty acids and infant development (editorial). *Lancet* 1999;354:1919.

59. Moriguchi T, Greiner RS, Salem N Jr. Behavioral deficits associated with dietary induction of decreased brain docosahexaenoic acid concentration. *J Neurochem* 2000;75:2563–2573.

60. Liu Z, Wang D, Xue Q, Chen J, Li Y, Bai X, Chang L. Determination of fatty acid levels in erythrocyte membranes of patients with chronic fatigue syndrome. *Nutr Neurosci* December 2003;6(6):389–392.

61. Gray JB, Martinovic AM. Eicosanoids and essential fatty acid modulation in chronic disease and the chronic fatigue syndrome. *Med Hypotheses* July 1994;43(1):31–42.

62. Horrobin DF. Post-viral fatigue syndrome, viral infections in atopic eczema, and essential fatty acids. *Med Hypotheses* 1990;32:211–217.

63. Gray JB, Martinovic AM. Eicosanoids and essential fatty acid modulation in chronic disease and the chronic fatigue syndrome. *Med Hypotheses.* July 1994;43(1):31–42.

64. Puri BK. Long-chain polyunsaturated fatty acids and the pathophysiology of myalgic encephalomyelitis (chronic fatigue syndrome). *J Clin Pathol* February 2007;60(2):122–124. Epub 2006 Aug 25.

65. Puri BK, Holmes J, Hamilton G. Eicosapentaenoic acid-rich essential fatty acid supplementation in chronic fatigue syndrome associated with symptom remission and structural brain changes. *Int J Clin Pract* March 2004;58(3):297–299.

66. Behan PO, Behan WM, Horrobin D. Effect of high doses of essential fatty acids on the postviral fatigue syndrome. *Acta Neurol Scand* September 1990;82(3):209–216.

67. Maes M, Mihaylova I, Leunis JC. In chronic fatigue syndrome, the decreased levels of omega-3 poly-unsaturated fatty acids are related to lowered serum zinc and defects in T cell activation. *Neuro Endocrinol Lett* December 2005;26(6):745–751.

68. Suitor CW, Bailey LB. Dietary folate equivalents: Interpretation and application. *J Am Diet Assoc* 2000;100:88–94.

69. Gregory JF. Case study: Folate bioavailability. *J Nutr* 2001;131:1376S–1382S.

70. Koebnick C, Heins UA, Hoffmann I, Dagnelie PC, Leitzmann C. Folate status during pregnancy in women is improved by long-term high vegetable intake compared with the average western diet. *J Nutr* 2001;131:733–739.

71. Selhub J, Jacques PF, Bostom AG, Wilson PW, Rosenberg IH. Relationship between plasma homocysteine and vitamin status in the Framingham study population. Impact of folic acid fortification. *Publ Health Rev* 2000;28:117–145.

72. Mayer O Jr, Simon J, Rosolová H, Hromádka M, Subrt I, Vobrubová I. The effects of folate supplementation on some coagulation parameter and oxidative status surrogates. *Eur J Clin Pharmacol* 2002;58:1–5.

73. Botez MI, Fontaine F, Botez T, Bachevalier J. Neuropsychological correlates of folic acid deficiency: facts and hypotheses. In: Botez MI, Reynolds EH, eds. *Folic acid in neurology, psychiatry, and internal medicine.* New York: Raven Press, 1979:435–461.

74. Godfrey P, Crellin R, Toone BK, Flynn TG, Carney MW, Laundy M, Chanarin I, Bottiglieri T, Reynolds EH. Enhancement of recovery from psychiatric illness by methylfolate. *Lancet* 1990;336:392–395.

75. Jacobson W, Saich T, Borysiewicz LK, Behan WM, Behan PO, Wreghitt TG. Serum folate and chronic fatigue syndrome. *Neurology* 1993;43:2645–2647.

76. Werbach MR. Nutritional strategies for treating chronic fatigue syndrome. *Altern Med Rev* April 2000;5(2):93–108.

77. Mayer EL, Jacobsen DW, Robinson K. Homocysteine and coronary atherosclerosis. *J Am Coll Cardiol* 1996;27:517–527.

78. Carmel R. Approach to a low vitamin B12 level. *JAMA* 1994;272:1233.

79. Regland B, Andersson M, Abrahamsson L, Bagby J, Dyrehag LE, Gottfries CG. Increased concentrations of homocysteine in the cerebrospinal fluid in patients with fibromyalgia and chronic fatigue syndrome. *Scand J Rheumatol* 1997;26:301–307.

80. Ellis FR, Nasser S. A pilot study of vitamin B12 in the treatment of tiredness. *Br J Nutr* 1973;30:277–283.

81. Newbold HL. Vitamin B-12: Placebo or neglected therapeutic tool? *Med Hypotheses* 1989;28:155–164.

82. Lapp CW, Cheney PR. The rationale for using high-dose cobalamin (Vitamin B12). The CFIDS Chronicle Physicians' Forum Fall 1993;19–20. CW Lapp, Q: Given the complexities and diversity of symptoms of CFIDS, how do you approach the treatment of CFIDS patients? The CFIDS Chronicle Physicians' Forum March 1991;1(1)

83. Kaslow JE, Rucker L, Onishi R. Liver extractfolic acid-cyanocobalamin vs placebo for chronic fatigue syndrome. *Arch Intern Med* 1989;149:2501–2503.

84. Mukherjee TM, Smith K, Maros K. Abnormal red-blood-cell morphology in myalgic encephalomyelitis. *Lancet* 1987;2:328–329.

85. Simpson LO. Nondiscocytic erythrocytes in myalgic encephalomyelitis. *N Z Med J* 1989;102:126–127.

86. Simpson LO, Murdoch JC, Herbison GP. Red cell shape changes following trigger finger fatigue in subjects with chronic tiredness and healthy controls. *N Z Med J* 1993;106:104–107.

87. Buist R. Elevated xenobiotics, lactate and pyruvate in C.F.S. patients. *J Orthomol Med* 1989;4:170–172.

88. Simpson LO. Myalgic encephalomyelitis. Letter. *J R Soc Med* 1991;84:633.

89. Heap LC, Peters TJ, Wessely S. Vitamin B status in patients with chronic fatigue syndrome. *J R Soc Med* 1999;92:183–185.

90. Grant JE, Veldee MS, Buchwald D. Analysis of dietary intake and selected nutrient concentrations in patients with chronic fatigue syndrome. *J Am Diet Assoc* 1996;96:383–386.

91. Shils ME, Olson JA, Shike M, Ross AC, eds. *Modern nutrition in health and disease.* 9th edn. Baltimore, MD: Williams & Wilkins, 1999.

92. Wolfe ML, Vartanian SF, Ross JL, Bansavich LL, Mohler ER 3rd, Meagher E, Friedrich CA, Rader DJ. Safety and effectiveness of Niaspan when added sequentially to a statin for treatment of dyslipidemia. *Am J Cardiol* 2001;87:476–479, A7.

93. Johansson JO, Egberg N, Asplund-Carlson A, Carlson LA. Nicotinic acid treatment shifts the fibrinolytic balance favourably and decreases plasma fibrinogen in hypertriglyceridaemic men. *J Cardiovasc Risk* 1997;4:165–171.

94. Birkmayer GD, Kay GG, Vurre E. [Stabilized NADH (ENADA) improves jet lag-induced cognitive performance deficit.] *Wien Med Wochenschr* 2002;152:450–454.

95. Forsyth LM, Preuss HG, MacDowell AL, Chiazze L Jr, Birkmayer GD, Bellanti JA. Therapeutic effects of oral NADH on the symptoms of patients with chronic fatigue syndrome. *Ann Allergy Asthma Immunol* 1999;82:185–191.

96. Santaella ML, Font I, Disdier OM. Comparison of oral nicotinamide adenine dinucleotide (NADH) versus conventional therapy for chronic fatigue syndrome. *P R Health J Sci* June 2004;23(2):89–93.

97. Lenzi A, Sgrò P, Salacone P, Paoli D, Gilio B, Lombardo F, Santulli M, Agarwal A, Gandini L. A placebo-controlled double-blind randomized trial of the use of combined l-carnitine and l-acetyl-carnitine treatment in men with asthenozoospermia. *Fertil Steril* 2004;81:1578–1584.

98. Liu J, Head E, Kuratsune H, Cotman CW, Ames BN. Comparison of the effects of L-carnitine and acetyl-L-carnitine on carnitine levels, ambulatory activity, and oxidative stress biomarkers in the brain of old rats. *Ann N Y Acad Sci* 2004;1033:117–131.

99. Stanley CA. Carnitine deficiency disorders in children. *Ann N Y Acad Sci* 2004;1033:42–51.

100. Berthillier G, Eichenberger D, Carrier HN, Guibaud P, Got R. Carnitine metabolism in early stages of Duchenne muscular dystrophy. *Clin Chim Acta* 1982;122:369–375.

101. Goral S. Levocarnitine and muscle metabolism in patients with end-stage renal disease. *J Ren Nutr* 1998;8:118–121.

102. Kletzmayr J, Mayer G, Legenstein E, Heinz-Peer G, Leitha T, Hörl WH, Kovarik J. Anemia and carnitine supplementation in hemodialyzed patients. *Kidney Int* 1999;69:93–106.

103. Hurot JM, Cucherat M, Haugh M, Fouque D. Effects of L-carnitine supplementation in maintenance hemodialysis patients: A systematic review. *J Am Soc Nephrol* 2002;13:708–714.

104. Moretti S. Effect of L-carnitine on human immunodeficiency virus-1 infection-associated apoptosis: a pilot study. *Blood* 1998;91:3817–3824.

105. Mintz M. Carnitine in human immunodeficiency virus type 1 infection/acquired immune deficiency syndrome. *J Child Neurol* 1995;10:S40–S44.

106. Plioplys AV, Plioplys S. Amantadine and L-carnitine treatment of chronic fatigue syndrome. *Neuropsychobiology* 1997;35:16–23.

107. Kuratsune H, Yamaguti K, Lindh G, Evengard B, Takahashi M, Machii T, Matsumura K, Takaishi J, Kawata S, Långström B, Kanakura Y, Kitani T, Watanabe Y. Low levels of serum acylcarnitine in chronic fatigue syndrome and chronic hepatitis type C, but not seen in other diseases. *Int J Mol Med* July 1998;2(1):51–56.

108. Kuratsune H, Yamaguti K, Takahashi M. Acylcarnitine deficiency in chronic fatigue syndrome. *Clin-Infect-Dis* January 1994;18 (Suppl 1) S62–S67.

109. Turunen M, Olsson J, Dallner G. Metabolism and function of coenzyme Q. *Biochim Biophys Acta* 2004;1660:171–199.

110. Chan A, Reichmann H, Kögel A, Beck A, Gold R. Metabolic changes in patients with mitochondrial myopathies and effects of coenzyme Q10 therapy. *J Neurol* 1998;245:681–685.

111. Chen RS, Huang CC, Chu NS. Coenzyme Q10 treatment in mitochondrial encephalomyopathies. Short-term double-blind, crossover study. *Eur Neurol* 1997;37:212–218.

112. Bresolin N, Doriguzzi C, Ponzetto C, Angelini C, Moroni I, Castelli E, Cossutta E, Binda A, Gallanti A, Gabellini S. Ubidecarenone in the treatment of mitochondrial myopathies: A multi-center double-blind trial. *J Neurol Sci* 1990;100:70–78.

113. Greenberg S, Fishman WH. Coenzyme Q10: A new drug for cardiovascular disease. *J Clin Pharmacol* 1990;30:596–608.

114. Bertelli A, Ronca G. Carnitine and coenzyme Q10: Biochemical properties and functions, synergism and complementary action. *Int J Tissue React* 1990;12:183–186.

115. Bertelli A, Cerrati A, Giovannini L, Mian M, Spaggiari P, Bertelli AA. Protective action of L-carnitine and coenzyme Q10 against hepatic triglyceride infiltration induced by hyperbaric oxygen and ethanol. *Drugs Exp Clin Res* 1993;19:65–68.

116. Crane FL. Biochemical functions of coenzyme Q10. *J Am Coll Nutr* 2001;20:591–598.

117. Matthews RT, Yang L, Browne S, Baik M, Beal MF. Coenzyme Q10 administration increases brain mitochondrial concentrations and exerts neuroprotective effects. *Proc Natl Acad Sci U S A* 1998;95:8892–8897.

118. McGroarty JA. Probiotic use of lactobacilli in the human female urogenital tract. *FEMS Immunol Med Microbiol* 1993;6:251–264.

119. Bruce AW, Reid G. Intravaginal instillation of Lactobacilli for prevention of recurrent urinary tract infections. *Can J Microbiol* 1988;34:339–343.

120. Madsen KL, Doyle JS, Jewell LD, Tavernini MM, Fedorak RN. Lactobacillus species prevents colitis in interleukin 10 gene-deficient mice. *Gastroenterology* 1999;116:1107–1114.

121. Casas IA, Dobrogosz WJ. Validation of the probiotic concept: Lactobacillus reuteri confers broad-spectrum protection against disease in humans and animals. *Microb Ecol Health Dis* 2000;12:247–285.

122. Shornikova AV, Casas IA, Isolauri E, Mykkänen H, Vesikari T. Lactobacillus reuteri as a therapeutic agent in acute diarrhea in young children. *J Pediatr Gastroenterol Nutr* 1997;24:399–404.

123. Alander M, Satokari R, Korpela R, Saxelin M, Vilpponen-Salmela T, Mattila-Sandholm T, von Wright A. Persistence of colonization of human colonic mucosa by a probiotic strain, Lactobacillus rhamnosus GG, after oral consumption. *Appl Environ Microbiol* 1999;65:351–354.

124. Sullivan A, Barkholt L, Nord CE. Lactobacillus acidophilus, Bifidobacterium lactis and Lactobacillus F19 prevent antibiotic-associated ecological disturbances of Bacteroides fragilis in the intestine. *J Antimicrob Chemother* 2003;52:308–311.

125. Madsen KL, Doyle JS, Jewell LD, Tavernini MM, Fedorak RN. Lactobacillus species prevents colitis in interleukin 10 gene-deficient mice. *Gastroenterology* 1999;116:1107–1114.

126. Vanderhoof JA, Young RJ. Current and potential uses of probiotics. *Ann Allergy Asthma Immunol* 2004;93:S33–S37.

127. Casas IA, Dobrogosz WJ. Validation of the probiotic concept: Lactobacillus reuteri confers broad-spectrum protection against disease in humans and animals. *Microb Ecol Health Dis* 2000;12:247–285.

128. Rautava S, Kalliomaki M, Isolauri E. Probiotics during pregnancy and breast-feeding might confer immunomodulatory protection against atopic disease in the infant. *J Allergy Clin Immunol* 2002;109:119–121.

129. Majamaa H, Isolauri E. Probiotics: A novel approach in the management of food allergy. *J Allergy Clin Immunol* 1997;99:179–185.

130. Olivares M, Paz Díaz-Ropero M, Gómez N, Sierra S, Lara-Villoslada F, Martín R, Miguel Rodríguez J, Xaus J. Dietary deprivation of fermented foods causes a fall in innate immune response. Lactic acid bacteria can counteract the immunological effect of this deprivation. *J Dairy Res* November 2006;73(4):492–498. Epub 2006 Sep 21.

131. Gackowska L, Michalkiewicz J, Krotkiewski M, Helmin-Basa A, Kubiszewska I, Dzierzanowska D. Combined effect of different lactic acid bacteria strains on the mode of cytokines pattern expression in human peripheral blood mononuclear cells. *J Physiol Pharmacol* November 2006;57(Suppl 9):13–21.

132. Alonso L, Cuesta EP, Gilliland SE. Production of free conjugated linoleic acid by Lactobacillus acidophilus and Lactobacillus casei of human intestinal origin. *J Dairy Sci.* June 2003;86(6):1941–1946.

133. Lin MY, Chang FJ. Antioxidative effect of intestinal bacteria Bifidobacterium longum ATCC 15708 and Lactobacillus acidophilus ATCC 4356. *Dig Dis Sci.* August 2000;45(8):1617–1622.

134. Logan AC, Wong C. Chronic fatigue syndrome: Oxidative stress and dietary modifications. *Altern Med Rev* October 2001;6(5):450–459.

135. Saxelin M. Colonization of the human gastrointestinal tract by probiotic bacteria (Lactobacillus GG). *Nutr Today* 1996;31:5S–8S.

CHAPTER 9

1. Singh A, Garg V, Gupta S, Kulkarni SK. Role of antioxidants in chronic fatigue syndrome in mice. *Indian J Exp Biol* November 2002;40(11):1240–1244.

2. Singh A, Naidu PS, Gupta S, Kulkarni SK. Effect of natural and synthetic antioxidants in a mouse model of chronic fatigue syndrome. *J Med Food* Winter 2002;5(4):211–220.

3. DerMarderosian A, Liberti L, Beutler JA, Grauds C. *The review of natural products published by facts and comparisons*. St. Louis, MO: Wolters Kluwer Co., 1999.

4. Cignarella A, Nastasi M, Cavalli E, Puglisi L. Novel lipid-lowering properties of Vaccinium myrtillus L. leaves, a traditional antidiabetic treatment, in several models of rat dyslipidaemia: A comparison with ciprofibrate. *Thromb Res* 1996;84:311–322.

5. Fraisse D, Carnat A, Lamaison JL. Polyphenolic composition of the leaf of bilberry. Article in French. *Ann Pharm Fr* 1996;54:280–283.

6. Wichtl MW. *Herbal drugs and phytopharmaceuticals*. In: NM Bisset ed. Stuttgart: Medpharm GmbH Scientific Publishers, 1994.

7. Wang SY, Jiao H. Scavenging capacity of berry crops on superoxide radicals, hydrogen peroxide, hydroxyl radicals, and singlet oxygen. *J Agric Food Chem* 2000;48:5677–5684.

8. Cao G, Shukitt-Hale B, Bickford PC, Joseph JA, McEwen J, Prior RL. Hyperoxia-induced changes in antioxidant capacity and the effect of dietary antioxidants. *J Appl Physiol* 1999;86:1817–1822.

9. Bickford PC, Gould T, Briederick L, Chadman K, Pollock A, Young D, Shukitt-Hale B, Joseph J. Antioxidant-rich diets improve cerebellar physiology and motor learning in aged rats. *Brain Res* 2000;866:211–217.

10. Cignarella A, Nastasi M, Cavalli E, Puglisi L. Novel lipid-lowering properties of Vaccinium myrtillus L. leaves, a traditional antidiabetic treatment, in several models of rat dyslipidaemia: A comparison with ciprofibrate. *Thromb Res* 1996;84:311–322.

11. Cao G, Booth SL, Sadowski JA, Prior RL. Increases in human plasma antioxidant capacity after consumption of controlled diets high in fruit and vegetables. *Am J Clin Nutr* 1998;68:1081–1087.

12. Cao G, Sofic E, Prior RL. Antioxidant capacity of tea and common vegetables. *J Agric Food Chem* 1996;44:3426–3431.

13. Wang H, Cao G, Prior RL. Total antioxidant capacity of fruits. *J Agric Food Chem* 1996;44:701–705.

14. Prior RL, Gu L, Wu X, Jacob RA, Sotoudeh G, Kader AA, Cook RA. Antioxidant capacity as influenced by total phenolic and anthocyanin content, maturity, and variety of Vaccinium species. *J Agric Food Chem* 1998;46:2686–2693.

15. Youdim KA, Shukitt-Hale B, MacKinnon S, Kalt W, Joseph JA. Polyphenolics enhance red blood cell resistance to oxidative stress: In vitro and in vivo. *Biochim Biophys Acta* 2000;1523:117–122.

16. Edwards AM, Blackburn L, Christie S. Food supplements in the treatment of fibromyalgia: A double-blind, crossover trial of anthocyanidins and placebo. *J Nutr Environ Med* 2000;10:189–199.

17. Perossini M, Guidi G, Chiellini S, Siravo D. Diabetic and hypertensive retinopathy therapy with Vaccinium myrtillus anthocyanosides (Tegens). Double blind, placebo-controlled clinical trial. Article in Italian. *Ann Ottalmol Clin Ocul* 1987;113:1173–1177.

18. Newall CA, Anderson LA, Philpson JD. *Herbal medicine: A guide for healthcare professionals.* London, UK: The Pharmaceutical Press, 1996.

19. Wichtl MW. *Herbal drugs and phytopharmaceuticals.* In: NM Bisset ed. Stuttgart: Medpharm GmbH Scientific Publishers, 1994.

20. McGuffin M, Hobbs C, Upton R, Goldberg A, eds. *American herbal products association's botanical safety handbook.* Boca Raton, FL: CRC Press, LLC, 1997.

21. Wu X, Cao G, Prior RL. Absorption and metabolism of anthocyanins in elderly women after consumption of elderberry or blueberry. *J Nutr* 2002;132:1865–1871.

22. Cao G, Prior RL. Anthocyanins are detected in human plasma after oral administration of an elderberry extract. *Clin Chem* 1999;45:574–576.

23. Zakay-Rones Z, Thom E, Wollan T, Wadstein J. Randomized study of the efficacy and safety of oral elderberry extract in the treatment of influenza A and B virus infections. *J Int Med Res* 2004;32:132–140.

24. Barak V, Halperin T, Kalickman I. The effect of Sambucol, a black elderberry-based, natural product, on the production of human cytokines: I. Inflammatory cytokines. *Eur Cytokine Netw* 2001;12:290–296.

25. Zakay-Rones Z, Thom E, Wollan T, Wadstein J. Inhibition of several strains of influenza virus in vitro and reduction of symptoms by an elderberry extract (Sambucus nigra L.) during an outbreak of influenza B Panama. *J Altern Complement Med* 1995;1:361–369.

26. Foster S, Hobbs C. *Western medicinal plants and herbs*, Peterson's Field Guide 2002. Boston: Houghton Mifflin Company.

27. Chevallier A. *The encyclopedia of medicinal plants.* London, UK: Dorling Kindersley, Ltd, 1996.

28. Bagchi D, Bagchi M, Stohs SJ, Das DK, Ray SD, Kuszynski CA, Joshi SS, Pruess HG. Free radicals and grape seed proanthocyanidin extract: Importance in human health and disease prevention. *Toxicology* 2000;148:187–197.

29. Meyer AS, Yi OS, Pearson DA. Inhibition of human low-density lipoprotein oxidation in relation to composition of phenolic antioxidants in grapes (Vitis vinifera). *J Agric Food Chem* 1997;45:1638–1643.

30. Chisholm A, Mc Auley K, Mann J, Williams S, Skeaff M. A diet rich in walnuts favourably influences plasma fatty acid profile in moderately hyperlipidaemic subjects. *Eur J Clin Nutr* 1998;52:12–16.

31. Freedman JE, Parker C 3rd, Li L, Perlman JA, Frei B, Ivanov V, Deak LR, Iafrati MD, Folts JD. Select flavonoids and whole juice from purple grapes inhibit platelet function and enhance nitric oxide release. *Circulation* 2001;103:2792–2798.

32. Nuttall SL, Kendall MJ, Bombardelli E, Morazzoni P. An evaluation of the antioxidant activity of a standardized grape seed extract, Leucoselect. *J Clin Pharm Ther* 1998;23:385–389.

33. Pataki T, Bak I, Kovacs P, Bagchi D, Das DK, Tosaki A. Grape seed proanthocyanidins improved cardiac recovery during reperfusion after ischemia in isolated rat hearts. *Am J Clin Nutr* 2002;75:894–899.

34. Stein JH, Keevil JG, Wiebe DA, Aeschlimann S, Folts JD. Purple grape juice improves endothelial function and reduces the susceptibility of LDL cholesterol to oxidation in patients with coronary artery disease. *Circulation* 1999;100:1050–1055.

35. Bagchi D, Bagchi M, Stohs S, Ray SD, Sen CK, Preuss HG. Cellular protection with proanthocyanidins derived from grape seeds. *Ann N Y Acad Sci* 2002;957:260–270.

36. Adcocks C, Collin P, Buttle DJ. Catechins from green tea (Camellia sinensis) inhibit bovine and human cartilage proteoglycan and type II collagen degradation in vitro. *J Nutr* 2002;132:341–346.

37. Haqqi TM, Anthony DD, Gupta S, Ahmad N, Lee MS, Kumar GK, Mukhtar H. Prevention of collagen-induced arthritis in mice by a polyphenolic fraction from green tea. *Proc Natl Acad Sci U S A* 1999;96:4524–4529.

38. Gupta S, Saha B, Giri AK. Comparative antimutagenic and anticlastogenic effects of green tea and black tea: A review. *Mutat Res* 2002;512:37–65.

39. Garbisa S, Biggin S, Cavallarin N, Sartor L, Benelli R, Albini A. Tumor invasion: Molecular shears blunted by green tea. *Nat Med* 1999;5:1216.

40. Cao Y, Cao R. Angiogenesis inhibited by drinking tea. *Nature* 1999;398:381.

41. L'Allemain G. Multiple actions of EGCG, the main component of green tea. Article in French. *Bull Cancer* 1999;86:721–724.

42. Pisters KM, Newman RA, Coldman B, Shin DM, Khuri FR, Hong WK, Glisson BS, Lee JS. Phase I trial of oral green tea extract in adult patients with solid tumors. *J Clin Oncol* 2001;19:1830–1838.

43. Kemberling JK, Hampton JA, Keck RW, Gomez MA, Selman SH. Inhibition of bladder tumor growth by the green tea derivative epigallocatechin-3-gallate. *J Urol* 2003;170:773–776.

44. Elmets CA, Singh D, Tubesing K, Matsui M, Katiyar S, Mukhtar H. Cutaneous photoprotection from ultraviolet injury by green tea polyphenols. *J Am Acad Dermatol* 2001;44:425–432.

45. Dulloo AG, Duret C, Rohrer D, Girardier L, Mensi N, Fathi M, Chantre P, Vandermander J. Efficacy of a green tea extract rich in catechin polyphenols and caffeine in increasing 24-h energy expenditure and fat oxidation in humans. *Am J Clin Nutr* 1999;70:1040–1045.

46. Cronin JR. Green tea extract stokes thermogenesis: Will it replace ephedra? *Altern Comp Ther* 2000;6:296–300.

47. Zheng G, Sayama K, Okubo T, Juneja LR, Oguni I. Anti-obesity effects of three major components of green tea, catechins, caffeine and theanine, in mice. *In Vivo* 2004;18:55–62.

48. Choi YT, Jung CH, Lee SR, Bae JH, Baek WK, Suh MH, Park J, Park CW, Suh SI. The green tea polyphenol (-)-epigallocatechin gallate attenuates beta-amyloid-induced neurotoxicity in cultured hippocampal neurons. *Life Sci* 2001;70:603–614.

49. Wu CH, Yang YC, Yao WJ, Lu FH, Wu JS, Chang CJ. Epidemiological evidence of increased bone mineral density in habitual tea drinkers. *Arch Intern Med* 2002;162:1001–1006.

50. Krahwinkel T, Willershausen B. The effect of sugar-free green tea chew candies on the degree of inflammation of the gingiva. *Eur J Med Res* 2000;5:463–467.

51. Katiyar SK, Afaq F, Perez A, Mukhtar H. Green tea polyphenol (-)-epigallocatechin-3-gallate treatment of human skin inhibits ultraviolet radiation-induced oxidative stress. Carcinogenesis. 2001 February;22(2):287–294.

52. Chung LY, Cheung TC, Kong SK, Fung KP, Choy YM, Chan ZY, Kwok TT. Induction of apoptosis by green tea catechins in human prostate cancer DU145 cells. *Life Sci* 2001;68:1207–1214.

53. Ahn WS, Yoo J, Huh SW, Kim CK, Lee JM, Namkoong SE, Bae SM, Lee IP. Protective effects of green tea extracts (polyphenon E and EGCG) on human cervical lesions. *Eur J Cancer Prev* 2003;12:383–390.

54. Leenen R, Roodenburg AJ, Tijburg LB, Wiseman SA. A single dose of tea with or without milk increases plasma antioxidant activity in humans. *Eur J Clin Nutr* 2000;54:87–92.

55. Hodgson JM, Puddey IB, Croft KD, Burke V, Mori TA, Caccetta RA, Beilin LJ. Acute effects of ingestion of black and green tea on lipoprotein oxidation. *Am J Clin Nutr* 2000;71:1103–1107.

56. Leung LK, Su Y, Chen R, Zhang Z, Huang Y, Chen ZY. Theaflavins in black tea and catechins in green tea are equally effective antioxidants. *J Nutr* 2001;131:2248–2251.

57. Weisburger JH. Tea and health: The underlying mechanisms. *Proc Soc Exp Biol Med* 1999;220:271–275.

58. Singal A, Kaur S, Tirkey N, Chopra K. Green tea extract and catechin ameliorate chronic fatigue-induced oxidative stress in mice. *J Med Food* Spring 2005;8(1):47–52.

59. Asmawi MZ, Kankaanranta H, Moilanen E, Vapaatalo H. Anti-inflammatory activities of Emblica officinalis Gaertn leaf extracts. *J Pharm Pharmacol* June 1993;45(6):581–584.

60. Vasudevan M. Parle M. Memory enhancing activity of Anwala churna (Emblica officinalis Gaertn.): An Ayurvedic preparation. *Physiol Behav* May 16, 2007;91(1):46–54. Epub February 8, 2007

61. Scartezzini P, Antognoni F, Raggi MA, Poli F, Sabbioni C. Vitamin C content and antioxidant activity of the fruit and of the Ayurvedic preparation of Emblica officinalis Gaertn. *J Ethnopharmacol* March 8, 2006;104(1–2):113–118. Epub October 13, 2005.

62. Rao TP, Sakaguchi N, Juneja LR, Wada E, Yokozawa T. Amla (Emblica officinalis Gaertn.) extracts reduce oxidative stress in streptozotocin-induced diabetic rats. *J Med Food* Fall 2005;8(3):362–368.

63. Naik GH, Priyadarsini KI, Bhagirathi RG, Mishra B, Mishra KP, Banavalikar MM, Mohan H. In vitro antioxidant studies and free radical reactions of triphala, an ayurvedic formulation and its constituents. *Phytother Res* July 2005;19(7):582–586.

64. Bhattacharya A, Ghosal S, Bhattacharya SK. Antioxidant activity of tannoid principles of Emblica officinalis (amla) in chronic stress induced changes in rat brain. *Indian J Exp Biol* September 2000;38(9):877–880.

65. Bhattacharya A, Chatterjee A, Ghosal S, Bhattacharya SK. Antioxidant activity of active tannoid principles of Emblica officinalis (amla). *Indian J Exp Biol* July 1999;37(7):676–680.

66. Damodaran M, Nair KR. A tannin from the Indian gooseberry (Phyllanthus emblica) with a protective action on ascorbic acid. *Biochem J* July 1936;30(6):1014–1020.

67. Yokozawa T, Kim YH, Kim JH, Okubo T, Chu DC, Juneja RL. Amla (Emblica officinalis Gaertn.) prevents dyslipidaemia and oxidative stress in the ageing process. *Br J Nutr* July 2007;97(6):1187–1195.

68. Suresh K, Vasudevan DM. Augmentation of murine natural killer cell and antibody dependent cellular cytotoxicity activities by Phyllanthus emblica, a new immunomodulator. *J Ethnopharmacol* August 1994;44(1):55–60.

69. Barrett B. Medicinal properties of Echinacea: A critical review. *Phytomedicine* 2003;10:66–86.

70. Luettig B, Steinmüller C, Gifford GE, Wagner H, Lohmann-Matthes ML. Macrophage activation by the polysaccharide arabinogalactan isolated from plant cell cultures of Echinacea purpurea. *J Natl Cancer Inst* 1989;81:669–675.

71. Stimpel M, Proksch A, Wagner H, Lohmann-Matthes ML. Macrophage activation and induction of macrophage cytotoxicity by purified polysaccharide fractions from the plant Echinacea purpurea. *Infect Immun* 1984;46:845–849.

72. Tragni E, Tubaro A, Melis S, Galli CL. Evidence from two classic irritation tests for an anti-inflammatory action of a natural extract, Echinacina B. *Food Chem Toxicol* 1985;23:317–319.

73. Müller-Jakic B, Breu W, Pröbstle A, Redl K, Greger H, Bauer R. In vitro inhibition of cyclooxygenase and 5-lipoxygenase by alkamides from Echinacea and Achillea species. *Planta Med* 1994;60:37–40.

74. See DM, Broumand N, Sahl L, Tilles JG. In vitro effects of echinacea and ginseng on natural killer and antibody-dependent cell cytotoxicity in healthy subjects and chronic fatigue syndrome or acquired immunodeficiency syndrome patients. *Immunopharmacology* January 1997;35(3):229–235.

75. Yale SH, Liu K. Echinacea purpurea therapy for the treatment of the common cold: A randomized, double-blind, placebo-controlled clinical trial. *Arch Intern Med* 2004;164:1237–1241.

76. Brinkeborn RM, Shah DV, Degenring FH. Echinaforce and other Echinacea fresh plant preparations in the treatment of the common cold. A randomized, placebo controlled, double-blind clinical trial. Phytomedicine. 1999 Mar;6(1):1–6.

77. Barrett B, Vohmann M, Calabrese C. Echinacea for upper respiratory infection. *J Fam Pract* 1999;48:628–635.

78. Lindenmuth GF, Lindenmuth EB. The efficacy of echinacea compound herbal tea preparation on the severity and duration of upper respiratory and flu symptoms: A randomized, double-blind, placebo-controlled study. *J Altern Complement Med* 2000;6:327–334.

79. Pepping J. Echinacea. *Am J Health Syst Pharm* 1999;56:121–123.

80. Upton R, ed. *Astragalus root: Analytical, quality control, and therapeutic monograph.* Santa Cruz, CA: American Herbal Pharmacopoeia, 1999:1–25.

81. McCulloch M, See C, Shu XJ, Broffman M, Kramer A, Fan WY, Gao J, Lieb W, Shieh K, Colford JM Jr. Astragalus-based Chinese herbs and platinum-based chemotherapy

for advanced non-small-cell lung cancer: Meta-analysis of randomized trials. *J Clin Oncol* 2006;24:419–430.

82. Shao BM, Xu W, Dai H, Tu P, Li Z, Gao XM. A study on the immune receptors for polysaccharides from the roots of Astragalus membranaceus, a Chinese medicinal herb. *Biochem Biophys Res Commun* 2004;320:1103–1111.

83. Sun Y, Hersh EM, Talpaz M, Lee SL, Wong W, Loo TL, Mavligit GM. Immune restoration and/or augmentation of local graft versus host reaction by traditional Chinese medicinal herbs. *Cancer* 1983;52:70–73.

84. Chu DT, Wong WL, Mavligit GM. Immunotherapy with Chinese medicinal herbs. I. Immune restoration of local xenogeneic graft-versus-host reaction in cancer patients by fractionated Astragalus membranaceus in vitro. *J Clin Lab Immunol* 1988;25:119–123.

85. Leung AY, Foster S. *Encyclopedia of common natural ingredients used in food, drugs and cosmetics.* 2nd edn. New York: John Wiley & Sons, 1996.

86. Upton R, ed. *Astragalus root: Analytical, quality control, and therapeutic monograph.* Santa Cruz, CA: American Herbal Pharmacopoeia, 1999:1–25.

87. Wasser SP, Weis AL. Therapeutic effects of substances occurring in higher Basidiomycetes mushrooms: A modern perspective. *Crit Rev Immunol* 1999;19:65–96.

88. Wang SY, Hsu ML, Hsu HC, Tzeng CH, Lee SS, Shiao MS, Ho CK. The antitumor effect of Ganoderma lucidum is mediated by cytokines released from activated macrophages and T lymphocytes. *Int J Cancer* 1997;70:699–705.

89. Gao Y, Zhou S, Jiang W, Huang M, Dai X. Effects of ganopoly (a Ganoderma lucidum polysaccharide extract) on the immune functions in advanced-stage cancer patients. *Immunol Invest* 2003;32:201–215.

90. Sun J, He H, Xie BJ. Novel antioxidant peptides from fermented mushroom Ganoderma lucidum. *J Agric Food Chem* 2004;52:6646–6652.

91. Aoki T, Usuda Y, Miyakoshi H, Tamura K, Herberman RB. Low natural killer syndrome: Clinical and immunological features. *Nat Immun Cell Growth Reg* 1987;6:116–128.

92. Miyakoshi H, Aoki T, Mizukoshi M. Acting mechanisms of lentinan in humans. II. Enhancement of non-specific cell-mediated cytotoxicity as an interferon-induced response. *Int J Immunopharmacol* 1984;6(4):373–379.

93. Blumenthal M, ed. *The complete German commission E monographs: therapeutic guide to herbal medicines.* Trans. S. Klein. Boston, MA: American Botanical Council, 1998.

94. Mur E, Hartig F, Eibl G, Schirmer M. Randomized double blind trial of an extract from the pentacyclic alkaloid-chemotype of uncaria tomentosa for the treatment of rheumatoid arthritis. *J Rheumatol* 2002;29:678–681.

95. Wurm M, Kacani L, Laus G, Keplinger K, Dierich MP. Pentacyclic oxindole alkaloids from Uncaria tomentosa induce human endothelial cells to release a lymphocyte-proliferation-regulating factor. *Planta Med* 1998;64:701–704.

96. Akesson Ch, Pero RW, Ivars F. C-Med 100, a hot water extract of Uncaria tomentosa, prolongs lymphocyte survival in vivo. *Phytomedicine* 2003;10:23–33.

97. Sandoval M, Charbonnet RM, Okuhama NN, Roberts J, Krenova Z, Trentacosti AM, Miller MJ. Cat's claw inhibits TNFalpha production and scavenges free radicals: Role in cytoprotection. *Free Radic Biol Med* 2000;29:71–78.

98. Piscoya J, Rodriguez Z, Bustamante SA, Okuhama NN, Miller MJ, Sandoval M. Efficacy and safety of freeze-dried cat's claw in osteoarthritis of the knee: Mechanisms of action of the species Uncaria guianensis. *Inflamm Res* 2001;50:442–448.

99. Lim TS, Na K, Choi EM, Chung JY, Hwang JK. Immunomodulating activities of polysaccharides isolated from Panax ginseng. *J Med Food* Spring 2004;7(1):1–6.

100. Scaglione F, Ferrara F, Dugnani S, Falchi M, Santoro G, Fraschini F. Immunomodulatory effects of two extracts of Panax ginseng CA Meyer. *Drugs Exp Clin Res* 1990;16:537–542.

101. McElhaney JE, Gravenstein S, Cole SK, Davidson E, O'neill D, Petitjean S, Rumble B, Shan JJ. A placebo-controlled trial of a proprietary extract of North American ginseng (CVT-E002) to prevent acute respiratory illness in institutionalized older adults. *J Am Geriatr Soc* 2004;52:13–19.

102. Wang M, Guilbert LJ, Li J, Wu Y, Pang P, Basu TK, Shan JJ. A proprietary extract from North American ginseng (Panax quinquefolium) enhances IL-2 and IFN-gamma productions in murine spleen cells induced by Con-A. *Int Immunopharmacol* 2004;4:311–315.

103. Luo P, Wang L. Peripheral blood mononuclear cell production of TNF-alpha in response to North American ginseng stimulation [abstract]. *Alt Ther* 2001;7:S21.

104. Wang M, Guilbert LJ, Li J, Wu Y, Pang P, Basu TK, Shan JJ. Immunomodulating activity of CVT-E002, a proprietary extract from North American ginseng (Panax quinquefolium). *J Pharm Pharmacol* 2001;53:1515–1523.

105. Kovacs K, Selye H. The original and creative scientist. *Ann NY Acad Sci* 1998;851:13–15.

106. Meletis C, Centrone W. Adrenal fatigue: Enhancing quality of life for patients with a functional disorder. *Alternative & Complementary Therapies* October 2002:267–272.

107. Davydov M, Krikorian AD. Eleutherococcus senticosus (Rupr. & Maxim.) Maxim. (Araliaceae) as an adaptogen: A closer look. *J Ethnopharmacol* 2000;72:345–393.

108. Han L, Cai D. Clinical and experimental study on treatment of acute cerebral infarction with Acanthopanax Injection. Article in Chinese. *Zhongguo Zhong Xi Yi Jie He Za Zhi* 1998;18:472–474.

109. Szolomicki S, Samochowiec L, Wojcicki J, Drozdzik M. The influence of active components of Eleutherococcus senticosus on cellular defense and physical fitness in man. *Phytother Res* 2000;14:30–35.

110. Bohn B, Nebe CT, Birr C. Flow-cytometric studies with Eleutherococcus senticosus extract as an immunomodulatory agent. *Arzneim Forsch* 1987;37:1193–1196.

111. Medon PJ, Ferguson PW, Watson CF. Effects of Eleutherococcus senticosus extracts on hexobarbital metabolism in vivo and in vitro. *J Ethnopharmacol* 1984;10:235–241.

112. Farnsworth NR, Awang DV, Waller DP, Martin AM. Siberian ginseng (Eleutherococcus senticosus): Current status as an adaptogen. *Econ Med Plant Res* 1985; 1:156–215.

113. Park HJ, Lee JH, Song YB, Park KH. Effects of dietary supplementation of lipophilic fraction from Panax ginseng on cGMP and cAMP in rat platelets and on blood coagulation. *Biol Pharm Bull* 1996;19:1434–1439.

114. Lewis R, Wake G, Court G, Court JA, Pickering AT, Kim YC, Perry EK. Non-ginsenoside nicotinic activity in ginseng species. *Phytother Res* 1999;13;59–64.

115. Tamaoki J, Nakata J, Kawatani K, Tagaya E, Nagai A. Ginsenoside-induced relaxation of human bronchial smooth muscle via release of nitric oxide. *Br J Pharmacol* 2000;130:1859–1864.

116. Shin HR, Kim JY, Yun TK, Morgan G, Vainio H. The cancer-preventive potential of Panax ginseng: A review of human and experimental evidence. *Cancer Causes Control* 2000;11:565–576.

117. Lee BM, Lee SK, Kim HS. Inhibition of oxidative DNA damage, 8-OHdG, and carbonyl contents in smokers treated with antioxidants (vitamin E, vitamin C, beta-carotene and red ginseng.) *Cancer Lett* 1998;132:219–227.

118. Kim YK, Guo Q, Packer L. Free radical scavenging activity of red ginseng aqueous extracts. *Toxicology* 2002;172:149–156.

119. Hiai S, Yokoyama H, Oura H, Yano S. Stimulation of pituitary-adrenocortical system by ginseng saponin. *Endocrinol Jpn* 1979;26:661–665.

120. Kase Y, Saitoh K, Ishige A, Komatsu Y. Mechanisms by which Hange-shashin-to reduces prostaglandin E2 levels. *Biol Pharm Bull* 1998;21:1277–1281.

121. Tode T, Kikuchi Y, Hirata J, Kita T, Nakata H, Nagata I. Effect of Korean red ginseng on psychological functions in patients with severe climacteric syndromes. *Int J Gynaecol Obstet* 1999;67:169–174.

122. Hikino H. Chapter 11: Traditional remedies and modern assessment: The case of ginseng. In: ROB Wijeskera ed. *The medicinal plant industry.* Boca Raton, FL: CRC Press, 1991: 149–166.

123. Shibata S. Chemistry and pharmacology of Panax. *Econ Med Plant Res* 1985;1:217–284.

124. Hallstrom C, Fulder S, Caruthers M. Effect of ginseng on the performance of nurses on night duty. *Comp Med East West* 1982;6:277–282.

125. Darbinyan V, Kteyan A, Panossian A, Gabrielian E, Wikman G, Wagner H. Rhodiola rosea in stress induced fatigue - a double blind cross-over study of a standardized extract SHR-5 with a repeated low-dose regimen on the mental performance of healthy physicians during night duty. *Phytomedicine* 2000;7:365–371.

126. Kelly GS. Rhodiola rosea: A possible plant adaptogen. *Altern Med Rev* 2001;6:293–302.

127. Panossian A, Wagner H. Stimulating effect of adaptogens: An overview with particular reference to their efficacy following single dose administration. *Phytother Res* October 2005;19(10):819–838.

128. Ha Z, Zhu Y, Zhang X, Cui J, Zhang S, Ma Y, Wang W, Jian X. The effect of rhodiola and acetazolamide on the sleep architecture and blood oxygen saturation in men living at high altitude. *Zhonghua Jie He He Hu Xi Za Zhi* September 2002;25(9):527–530.

129. Zhang Y, Liu Y. Study on effects of salidroside on lipid peroxidation on oxidative stress in rat hepatic stellate cells *Zhong Yao Cai* September 2005;28(9):794–796.

130. Kanupriya-Prasad D, Ram SM, Kumar R, Sawhney RC, Sharma SK. Ilavazhagan G, Kumar D, Banerjee PK. Cytoprotective and antioxidant activity of Rhodiola imbricata against tert-butyl hydroperoxide induced oxidative injury in U-937 human macrophages. *Mol Cell Biochem* July 2005;275(1–2):1–6.

131. Perfumi M, Mattioli L. Adaptogenic and central nervous system effects of single doses of 3% rosavin and 1% salidroside Rhodiola rosea L. extract in mice. *Phytother Res* January 2007;21(1):37–43.

132. De Bock K, Eijnde BO, Ramaekers M, Hespel P. Acute Rhodiola rosea intake can improve endurance exercise performance. *Int J Sport Nutr Exerc Metab* 2004;14:298–307.

133. Abidov M, Crendal F, Grachev S, Seifulla R, Ziegenfuss T. Effect of extracts from Rhodiola rosea and Rhodiola crenulata (Crassulaceae) roots on ATP content in mitochondria of skeletal muscles. *Bull Exp Biol Med* December 2003;136(6):585–587.

134. Shevtsov VA, Zholus BI, Shervarly VI, Vol'skij VB, Korovin YP, Khristich MP, Roslyakova NA, Wikman G. A randomized trial of two different doses of a SHR-5 rhodiola

rosea extract versus placebo and control of capacity for mental work. *Phytomedicine* March 2003;10, no.2–3 :95–105.

135. Petkov VD, Yonkov D, Mosharoff A, Kambourova T, Alova L, Petkov VV, Todorov I. Effects of alcohol aqueous extract from Rhodiola rosea L. roots on learning and memory. *Acta Physiol Pharmacol Bulg* 1986;12:3–16.

136. Spasov AA, Wikman GK, Mandrikov VB, Mironova IA, Neumoin VV. A double-blind, placebo-controlled pilot study of the stimulating and adaptogenic effect of Rhodiola rosea SHR-5 extract on the fatigue of students caused by stress during an examination period with a repeated low-dose regimen. *Phytomedicine* 2000;7:85–89.

137. Kumagai A, Nishino K, Shimomura A, Kin A, Yamamura Y. Effect of glycyrrhizin on estrogen action. *Endocrinol Jpn* 1967;14:34–38.

138. Parle M, Dhingra D, Kulkarni SK. Memory-strengthening activity of Glycyrrhiza glabra in exteroceptive and interoceptive behavioral models. *J Med Food* Winter 2004;7(4):462–466.

139. Demitrack MA. Chronic fatigue syndrome: A disease of the hypothalamic-pituitary-adrenal axis? *Ann Med* 1994;26:1–5.

140. De Becker P, De Meirleir K, Joos E, Campine I, Van Steenberge E, Smitz J, Velkeniers B. Dehydroepiandrosterone (DHEA) response to i.v. ACTH in patients with chronic fatigue syndrome. *Horm Metab Res* January 1999;31(1):18–21.

141. Whorwood CB, Sheppard MC, Stewart PM. Licorice inhibits 11 beta-hydroxysteroid dehydrogenase messenger ribonucleic acid levels and potentiates glucocorticoid hormone action. *Endocrinology* 1993;132:2287–2292.

142. Cleare AJ, Heap E, Malhi GS, Wessely S, O'Keane V, Miell J. Low-dose hydrocortisone in chronic fatigue syndrome: A randomised crossover trial. *Lancet* February 6, 1999;353(9151):455–458.

143. McKenzie R, O'Fallon A, Dale J, Demitrack M, Sharma G, Deloria M, Garcia-Borreguero D, Blackwelder W, Straus SE. Low-dose hydrocortisone for treatment of chronic fatigue syndrome: A randomized controlled trial. *JAMA* September 23–30, 1998;280(12):1061–1066.

144. Baschetti R. Chronic fatigue syndrome and liquorice. *N Z Med J* April 26, 1995;108(998):156–157.

145. Upton R, ed. *Ashwagandha root (Withania somnifera): Analytical, quality control, and therapuetic monograph.* Santa Cruz, CA: American Herbal Pharmacopoeia, 2000:1–25.

146. Davis L, Kuttan G. Effect of Withania somnifera on cyclophosphamide-induced urotoxicity. *Cancer Lett* 2000;148:9–17.

147. Archana R, Namasivayam A. Antistressor effect of Withania somnifera. *J Ethnopharmacol* 1999;64:91–93.

148. Bhattacharya SK, Satyan KS, Ghosal S. Antioxidant activity of glycowithanolides from Withania somnifera. *Indian J Exp Biol* 1997;35:236–239.

149. Mishra LC, Singh BB, Dagenais S. Scientific basis for the therapeutic use of Withania somnifera (ashwagandha): A review. *Altern Med Rev* 2000;5:334–346.

150. Ahmad M, Saleem S, Ahmad AS, Ansari MA, Yousuf S, Hoda MN, Islam F. Neuroprotective effects of Withania somnifera on 6-hydroxydopamine induced Parkinsonism in rats. *Hum Exp Toxicol* March 2005;24(3):137–147.

151. Sankar SR, Manivasagam T, Krishnamurti A, Ramanathan M. The neuroprotective effect of Withania somnifera root extract in MPTP-intoxicated mice: An analysis of behavioral and biochemical varibles. *Cell Mol Biol Lett* April 6, 2007 [Epub ahead of print].

152. Malik F, Singh J, Khajuria A, Suri KA, Satti NK, Singh S, Kaul MK, Kumar A, Bhatia A, Qazi GN. A standardized root extract of Withania somnifera and its major constituent withanolide-A elicit humoral and cell-mediated immune responses by up regulation of Th1-dominant polarization in BALB/c mice. *Life Sci* March 27, 2007;80(16):1525–1538. Epub January 25, 2007.

153. Davis L, Kuttan G. Suppressive effect of cyclophosphamide-induced toxicity by Withania somnifera extract in mice. *J Ethnopharmacol* 1998;62:209–214.

154. Bhattacharya SK, Muruganandam AV. Adaptogenic activity of Withania somnifera: An experimental study using a rat model of chronic stress. *Pharmacol Biochem Behav* June 2003;75(3):547–555.

155. Kuboyama T, Tohda C, Komatsu K. Neuritic regeneration and synaptic reconstruction induced by withanolide A. *Br J Pharmacol* April 2005;144(7):961–971.

156. Singh S. Mechanism of action of antiinflammatory effect of fixed oil of Ocimum basilicum Linn. *Indian J Exp Biol* March 1999;37(3):248–252.

157. Gupta SK, Prakash J, Srivastava S. Validation of traditional claim of Tulsi, Ocimum sanctum Linn. As a medicinal plant. *Indian J Exp Biol* July 2002;40(7):765–773.

158. Rai V, Iyer U, Mani UV. Effect of Tulasi (Ocimum sanctum) leaf powder supplementation on blood sugar levels, serum lipids and tissue lipids in diabetic rats. *Plant Foods Hum Nutr* 1997;50(1):9–16.

159. Sarkar A, Lavania SC, Pandey DN, Pant MC. Changes in the blood lipid profile after administration of Ocimum sanctum (Tulsi) leaves in the normal albino rabbits. *Indian J Physiol Pharmacol* October 1994;38(4):311–312.

160. Singh S, Majumdar DK. Evaluation of anti-inflammatory activity of fatty acids of Ocimum sanctum fixed oil. *Indian J Exp Bio* April 1997;35(4):380–383.

161. Devi PU, Ganasoundari A. Modulation of glutathione and antioxidant enzymes by Ocimum sanctum and its role in protection against radiation injury. *Indian J Exp Biol* March 1999;37(3):262–268.

162. Yanpallewar SU, Rai S, Kumar M, Acharya SB. Evaluation of antioxidant and neuroprotective effect of Ocimum sanctum on transient cerebral ischemia and long-term cerebral hypoperfusion. *Pharmacol Biochem Behav* September 2004;79(1):155–164.

163. Joshi H, Parle M. Evaluation of nootropic potential of Ocimum sanctum Linn. in mice. *Indian J Exp Biol* February 2006;44(2):133–136.

164. Maity TK, Mandal SC, Saha BP, Pal M. Effect of Ocimum sanctum roots extract on swimming performance in mice. *Phytother Res* March 2000;14(2):120–121.

165. Bhattacharya SK, Bhattacharya A, Chakrabarti A. Adaptogenic activity of Siotone, a polyherbal formulation of Ayurvedic rasayanas. *Indian J Exp Biol* February 2000;38(2):119–128.

166. Murch SJ, Simmons CB, Saxena PK. Melatonin in feverfew and other medicinal plants. *Lancet* 1997;350:1598–1599.

167. Laakmann G, Schule C, Baghai T, Kieser M. St. John's wort in mild to moderate depression: The relevance of hyperforin for the clinical efficacy. *Pharmacopsych* 1998;31:54–59.

168. Laakmann G, Schule C, Baghai T, Kieser M. St. John's wort in mild to moderate depression: The relevance of hyperforin for the clinical efficacy. *Pharmacopsych* 1998;31:54–59.

169. Jakovljević V, Popović M, Mimica-Dukić N, Sabo A, Gvozdenović L. Pharmacodynamic study of Hypericum perforatum L. *Phytomedicine* 2000;7:449–453.

170. Jensen AG, Hansen SH, Nielsen EO. Adhyperforin as a contributor to the effect of Hypericum perforatum L. in biochemical models of antidepressant activity. *Life Sci* 2001;68:1593–1605.

171. Müller WE, Singer A, Wonnemann M, Hafner U, Rolli M, Schäfer C. Hyperforin represents the neurotransmitter reuptake inhibiting constituent of hypericum extract. *Pharmacopsychiatry* 1998;31:16–21.

172. Kleber E, Obry T, Hippeli S, Schneider W, Elstner EF. Biochemical activities of extracts from Hypericum perforatum L. *Arzneimittelforschung* 1999;49:106–109.

173. Calapai G, Crupi A, Firenzuoli F, Inferrera G, Squadrito F, Parisi A, De Sarro G, Caputi A. Serotonin, norepinephrine and dopamine involvement in the antidepressant action of hypericum perforatum. *Pharmacopsychiatry* 2001;34:45–49.

174. Chatterjee SS, Noldner M, Koch E, Erdelmeier C. Antidepressant activity of hypericum perforatum and hyperforin: The neglected possibility. *Pharmacopsych* 1998;31:7–15.

175. Schule C, Baghai T, Ferrera A, Laakmann G. Neuroendocrine effects of Hypericum extract WS 5570 in 12 healthy male volunteers. *Pharmacopsychiatry* 2001;34:S127–S133.

176. Singer A, Wonnemann M, Muller WE. Hyperforin, a major antidepressant constituent of St. John's wort, inhibits serotonin uptake by elevating free intracellular Na+11. *J Pharmacol Exp Ther* 1999;290:1363–1368.

177. Jensen AG, Hansen SH, Nielsen EO. Adhyperforin as a contributor to the effect of Hypericum perforatum L. In biochemical models of antidepressant activity. *Life Sci* 2001;68:1593–1605.

178. Kumar V, Jaiswal AK, Singh PN, Bhattacharya SK. Anxiolytic activity of Indian Hypericum perforatum Linn: An experimental study. *Indian J Exp Biol* 2000;38:36–41.

179. Diamond BJ, Shiflett SC, Feiwel N, Matheis RJ, Noskin O, Richards JA, Schoenberger NE. Ginkgo biloba extract: Mechanisms and clinical indications. *Arch Phys Med Rehabil* 2000;81:668–678.

180. National Institutes of Health, *Clinical trials*. Available at: www.clinicaltrials.gov/ct/gui/c/r

181. Le Bars PL, Katz MM, Berman N, Itil TM, Freedman AM. Schatzberg AF. A placebo-controlled, double-blind, randomized trial of an extract of Ginkgo biloba for dementia. North American EGb Study Group. *JAMA* 1997;278:1327–1332.

182. Bastianetto S, Ramassamy C, Doré S, Christen Y, Poirier J, Quirion R. The ginkgo biloba extract (EGb 761) protects hippocampal neurons against cell death induced by beta-amyloid. *Eur J Neurosci* 2000;12:1882–1890.

183. Logani S, Chen MC, Tran T, Le T, Raffa RB. Actions of Ginkgo Biloba related to potential utility for the treatment of conditions involving cerebral hypoxia. *Life Sci* 2000;67:1389–1396.

184. Ranchon I, Gorrand JM, Cluzel J, Droy-Lefaix MT, Doly M. Functional protection of photoreceptors from light-induced damage by dimethylurea and Ginkgo biloba extract. *Invest Ophthalmol Vis Sci* 1999;40:1191–1199.

185. Brautigam MR, Blommaert FA, Verleye G. Treatment of age-related memory complaints with Gingko biloba extract: A randomized double blind placebo-controlled study. *Phytomedicine* 1998;5:425–434.

186. Kudolo GB. The effect of 3-month ingestion of Ginkgo biloba extract on pancreatic beta-cell function in response to glucose loading in normal glucose tolerant individuals. *J Clin Pharmacol* 2000;40:647–654.

187. Kudolo GB, Delaney D, Blodgett J. Short-term oral ingestion of Ginkgo biloba extract (EGb 761) reduces malondialdehyde levels in washed platelets of type 2 diabetic subjects. *Diabetes Res Clin Pract* 2005;68:29–38.

188. Allain H, Raoul P, Lieury A, LeCoz F, Gandon JM, d'Arbigny P. Effect of two doses of ginkgo biloba extract (EGb 761) on the dual-coding test in elderly subjects. *Clin Ther*. 1993 May-Jun;15(3):549–58.

189. Oken BS, Storzbach DM, Kaye JA. The efficacy of Ginkgo biloba on cognitive function in Alzheimer disease. *Arch Neurol* 1998;55:1409–1415.

190. DeFeudis FV, Drieu K. Ginkgo biloba extract (EGb 761) and CNS functions: basic studies and clinical applications. *Curr Drug Targets*. 2000 Jul;1(1):25–58.

191. Campos-Toimil M, Lugnier C, Droy-Lefaix MT. Takeda K. Inhibition of type 4 phosphodiesterase by rolipram and Ginkgo biloba extract (EGb 761) decreases agonist-induced rises in internal calcium in human endothelial cells. *Arterioscler Thromb Vasc Biol* 2000;20:e34–e40.

192. Heck AM, DeWitt BA, Lukes AL. Potential interactions between alternative therapies and warfarin. *Am J Health Syst Pharm* 2000;57:1221–1227.

193. Kudolo GB, Dorsey S, Blodgett J. Effect of the ingestion of Ginkgo biloba extract on platelet aggregation and urinary prostanoid excretion in healthy and Type 2 diabetic subjects. *Thromb Res* 2002;108:151–160.

194. Arenz A, Klein M, Fiehe K, Groß J, Drewke C, Hemscheidt T, Leistner E. Occurrence of neurotoxic 4'-O-methylpyridoxine in ginkgo biloba leaves, ginkgo medications and Japanese ginkgo food. *Planta Med* 1996;62:548–551.

195. Rigney U, Kimber S, Hindmarch I. The effects of acute doses of standardized Ginkgo biloba extract on memory and psychomotor performance in volunteers. *Phytother Res* 1999;13:408–415.

196. Subhan Z, Hindmarch I. The psychopharmacological effects of Ginkgo biloba extract in normal healthy volunteers. *Int J Clin Pharmacol Res* 1984;4:89–93.

197. Kennedy DO, Scholey AB, Wesnes KA. The dose-dependent cognitive effects of acute administration of Ginkgo biloba to healthy young volunteers. *Psychopharmacology (Berl)* 2000;151:416–423.

Index

About the Author and Series Editor

DAIVATI BHARADVAJ, N.D., is a Naturopathic Physician in private practice. A part-time faculty member at the National College of Naturopathic Medicine in Oregon, Bharadvaj is also a graduate of the college. Bharadvaj's undergraduate degree in nutritional sciences was earned at the Cornell University College of Human Ecology.

CHRIS D. MELETIS, N.D., is Senior Series Editor. He is the Executive Director for the Institute for Healthy Aging, www.TheIHA.org, a nonprofit organization dedicated to educating the public, media, and professional community on scientific approaches to enhancing healthy aging. He was chosen for the Naturopathic Physician of the Year Award for 2003–2004 by the American Association of Naturopathic Physicians. He is an international lecturer, a radio personality, and an educator of medical doctors, nurses, pharmacists, and the allied health care fields. He has authored ten books on natural health topics.